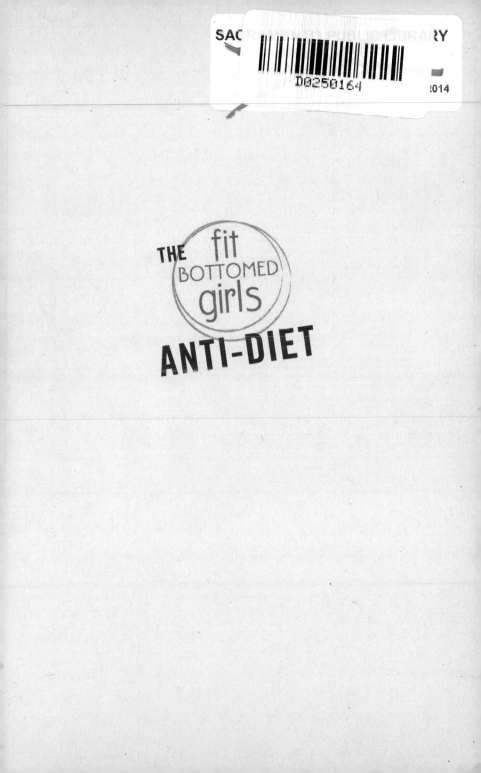

THE fit BOTTOMED girls
ANTI-DIET

THE 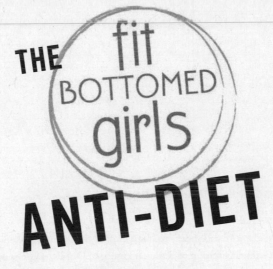 fit BOTTOMED girls ANTI-DIET

10-MINUTE FIXES TO GET THE BODY YOU WANT AND A LIFE YOU'LL LOVE

Jennipher Walters and Erin Whitehead

 HARMONY • NEW YORK

Published in the United States by Harmony Books, an imprint of the Crown Publishing Group, a division of Random House LLC, a Penguin Random House Company, New York. www.crownpublishing.com

Harmony Books is a registered trademark, and the Circle colophon is a trademark of Random House LLC.

Library of Congress Cataloging-in-Publication Data
Walters, Jennipher.
The fit bottomed girls anti-diet: 10-minute fixes to get the body you want and a life you'll love/by Jennipher Walters and Erin Whitehead.—First edition.
1. Women—Health and hygiene. 2. Weight training for women. 3. Body image in women. I. Whitehead, Erin. II. Title.
RA778.W2168 2013
613.7—dc23   2013032127

ISBN 978-0-8041-3697-6
eISBN 978-0-8041-3698-3

Printed in the United States of America

Book design by Kay Schuckhart/Blond on Pond

10 9 8 7 6 5 4 3 2 1

First Edition

To all of the FBG readers out there. You inspire us—
and truly make our rockin' world go round!

Contents

Introduction

....

Congrats! Knucks! Sparkle fingers! High five! Woo to the hoo!

Why exactly are we celebrating, you ask? Because you picked up this book! And in our experience, the hardest step in doing anything new is the *first* step. Maybe you're looking to lose some weight. Maybe you're tired of yo-yo dieting and obsessing about calories and the number on the scale. Maybe you're already a reader of our websites, FitBottomedGirls.com, FitBottomedMamas.com, and FitBottomedEats.com. Or, heck, maybe you're a Queen fan and the "Fat Bottomed Girl" song reference really rocked your world. (We couldn't really blame you there. We love a good homage to Queen, too.) No matter why you picked up this book, we are glad that you did. You're already one step closer to living a healthier, happier, and generally more awesome life.

We've been preaching for years that a healthy lifestyle isn't about deprivation or torturous workouts. Instead, it's about adding more fabulous stuff to your life. It's about doing the workouts you love, eating the healthy foods that make your taste buds do a happy dance, and treating yourself with the respect and self-love that you deserve. And then, from all that good stuff, you begin to feel awesome and allow that feel-good energy to create positive change in all areas of your life—not just the size of your pants. (Although that's certainly a perk.) It's not about depriving yourself or punishing yourself with nothing but carrots, grapefruit, and grueling gym sessions for the two weeks before your high school reunion to fit into that little black dress. It's about living well and feeling your best forever—and finding a healthy lifestyle that works for you and your life. And while that message has reached millions since the launch of our first site in May 2008, we've gotten greedy. We want to spread the word to every single woman (and dude, if you're a dude reading this book!) out there. We want to help you become your absolute best—and we want you to have a total blast while you're doing it.

On our websites, we talk a lot about "being an FBG," which includes picking workouts you love and eating according to your hunger; and it does *not* include letting the number on the scale determine your self-worth. But we never had a definitive guide on how to fully eat, work out, think, and live like a Fit Bottomed Girl, day after day. This, friends, is that guide. Based on our own experiences, our work with readers, and many hours researching what truly works and what doesn't, this book spells out exactly how to be a Fit Bottomed Girl, inside and out.

Now, this isn't designed to be a plan that you can knock out in two weeks and be done with, like so many of the diet books on the market. What we've put together is meant to help you transform your mindset about health and fitness in a lasting way. Like, in a *forever* way. Everyone wants the magic bullet or super-quick fix to getting healthy, but the real secret is that having a healthy life is founded on a good attitude and a love of that life. So, in order to change your life in that forever way, you have to set yourself up to enjoy your healthy eats and workouts and find the joy in it every day. You have to believe in yourself and believe that you're worth taking care of. That's why, chapter after chapter, you'll get doses of self-love, motivation, and plenty of ideas to inspire your healthy life. Instead of giving you a "diet" to try to stick to until you reach your goal, we'll help you create your ideal healthy life. In fact, our goal here is that these principles will become so ingrained that you won't even have to *try* to "be healthy" anymore. You just are. And it will feel amazing.

Again, this book is truly meant to give you a full body-mind-spirit life transformation. Because—news flash!—your health is about so much more than just your body. But instead of having you make a whole bunch of massive changes that totally disrupt your life—which, let's face it, will never last, no matter how good your intentions are—we're going to help you make itty-bitty adjustments that will become permanent fixtures. These small shifts may not seem like a big deal as you make them one by one, but over time they'll add up to great changes that stick. And that's what we want: for you to be a Fit Bottomed Girl not for just the next month but for life. Tiny change by tiny change, you'll begin to feel better, inside and out.

And the best part? By just reading this far, you've already come that much closer to reaching your healthy living dreams! So pat yourself on the butt—er, we mean back—and dive in!

What Is a Fit Bottomed Girl, Anyway?

Over the next ten chapters, we'll detail the principles that will allow you to achieve these awesome changes and to become the Fit Bottomed Girl we know you can be. We'll discuss how to eat, how to work out, how to treat your body, how to talk to yourself, and how to get and stay motivated. But before we get into those guidelines, let's break down what a Fit Bottomed Girl looks, acts, and feels like.

A Fit Bottomed Girl . . .

- Focuses her mental energy on what's really important in life
- Gets her self-confidence from within
- Listens to and honors her hunger
- Regularly does activities and workouts that she enjoys
- Eats everything in moderation
- Gets energy from feel-good workouts
- Talks to herself like she's her own best friend

It's equally important to bust down what an FBG *isn't*. And, spoiler alert: it has nothing to do with the size of your bum!

What a Fit Bottomed Girl Isn't . . .

- An obsessive calorie-counter
- Someone who lets the number on the scale determine her self-worth or mood for the day
- A meal-skipper
- Someone who uses exercise as punishment
- Someone who uses exercise to "burn off" foods

- Going to write off entire food groups
- At the gym for hours, forcing herself to do workouts she hates
- Her own worst enemy

Did you get all that? The "isn't"s are a lot of what many of us women have been trained to do to lose weight and "get healthy" over the years. But these methods don't work. You probably know that from experience. We certainly do. They are unhealthy behaviors that serve only to make you feel guilty, unworthy, and unsuccessful. Being obsessive about what you eat, beating yourself up for what you weigh, or feeling guilty about not getting to the gym every day is a surefire way to drain your self-confidence, which can carry over into all other areas of your life. When you spend all of your energy berating yourself for not being better, you're not going to have the energy left over to actually make changes that will help you reach your goals!

That's why being an FBG is about feeling in control of your life and your choices, rather than feeling as though your choices control your life. It's owning your decisions, being proud of who you are, and genuinely feeling good about how you use your body, no matter what the number on the scale reads. It's about respecting yourself, knowing that you deserve to live your best life, and tapping into your inner peace and happiness. As you read through the guidelines and progress through the book, keep this in mind: try being a Fit Bottomed Girl on for size. We think the FBG life will clearly be the more fulfilling path to be on. In fact, it's life-changingly awesome.

How to Use This Book

You may have picked up this anti-diet book because you wanted someone to tell you exactly what to do to get healthier. We understand—it's easy to get bogged down and overwhelmed by all the information out there, and it's easier to follow a strict plan. But do strict plans work for the long haul? Much like a cabbage soup diet can be "stomached" for only a day or two, it's unlikely that the average person can stick to a plan that has no wiggle room. Besides, we're more about having fun and less about being bossy around here, which is why we're not even going to tell you exactly how to use this book.

Here's what we've done. Each chapter is built upon an unbreakable rule for being a Fit Bottomed Girl. We share some concrete steps on how to tweak your lifestyle, from what you eat, to how you move, to how you talk to yourself. These small steps will add up to huge changes by the end of the program. Each chapter's 10-Minute Fixes include tweaks to your lifestyle—your diet, workouts, and even your way of thinking—that you can implement now to improve your life, as well as journaling exercises we promise will be time well spent. We've even got workout ideas and recipes to get you started. We also help you find new ways to feel better—and we can promise that there's no cabbage soup involved (unless you really do like the stuff; then, more power to you and your cabbage soup!).

If you like structure, you can treat each chapter as a lesson plan and spend a week taking it all in, focusing on that one area and adjusting parts of your lifestyle accordingly. If you'd rather pick and choose what works for you, this plan allows you that flexibility, too! We have a detailed Two-Week FBG Plan at the end of the book

WHAT'S WITH ALL THOSE SIDEBARS?

Each chapter has reoccurring sidebars—familiar friends who will visit you along your journey. The "From the FBGs" sidebars share our personal stories related to each of the principles and what we've learned along the way. We've been around the fitness, health, and body image block a time or two, so we hope our experiences can help you on your trip, too. Our "Energize" sidebars will have specific tips and tricks for finding energy all day, every day. Our "Fit Bottomed Mantras" throughout the book will give you those little motivational quotes and phrases to power you through the tough times—whether the tough times are on your couch conjuring up the motivation to get to the gym, during your last few squats at the gym, or trying to kick your negative thoughts to the curb.

on how to live the FBG life, with sample workouts and meals, but if you find one chapter zeros in on one of your particular trouble zones, feel free to linger there and explore. We won't tell you you're wrong. Promise.

The Power of 10 Minutes

Some diet plans promise big results over weeks and months. We can do better. We promise results in 10 minutes flat. Sure, that sounds like an infomercial. But we are certain that the 10-Minute Fixes you'll find in each chapter will have you more energized, fitter, healthier, and happier by the time you're finished with the first one!

We know how daunting it can be when you hear the recommendations for exercise and healthy eating. You're busy already;

how on earth can you fit in an hour of exercise? How can you find time to cook a healthy meal when you have kids and an hour-long commute? *But everyone has 10 minutes.* Heck, you probably spend 10 minutes mindlessly surfing the Internet or watching TV every day. And the good news is that we're not telling you to put down the remote control; you can do a lot of these 10-minute changes *while* you're online or catching up on your favorite shows! You'll be surprised at how little time and effort it takes to make healthy adjustments to your lifestyle—and you may even start to like it! (In fact, we're betting that you will.) You'll start to think of these changes as something positive you're adding to your life instead of the deprivation that so many diets require. We're not about deprivation—deprivation is sad and restrictive, and it's not sustainable. Once you see some of the fun things you can add into your life, you'll never want to go back!

ENERGIZE!
The Power of a Smile

Need an instant pick-me-up? Put down that coffee cup and turn that frown upside down! The clichés "fake it 'til you make it" and "grin and bear it"—they're actually rooted in smile psychology. Turns out, when you smile, your facial muscles send signals to your brain, letting it know what emotions you're feeling. Studies suggest that simply flashing a smile can give your mood a boost, and it can also help you recover from stressors. Even relaxing your face—like when you're eking out that last push-up—can help control your emotions. So flash that toothy grin and feel the effects on your psyche. It takes more muscles to frown than it does to smile, but this is one time we actually advocate working fewer muscles!

Don't think 10 minutes is enough time to do anything? We'll prove you wrong. Throughout the book we've provided dozens of 10-Minute Fixes, or tricks, to get you on the path to success—from fast ideas for healthy meals, to super-quick workouts, to tweaks for better sleep. Remember how we said that sometimes the first step is the hardest? Our 10-Minute Fixes help to make those steps feel like something you will actually be able to do. They're manageable and fun—and they'll set you up for success. And once some of these new habits take hold, you'll start to see the benefits and want to add more. It's a health spiral!

Now, Let's Do This!

By now, we hope we've convinced you that being a Fit Bottomed Girl is pretty rad. And as you go through each principle, you'll begin to feel that in your body and soul. Because, truly, becoming a Fit Bottomed Girl is about more than just being at a healthy weight, eating right, and working out. It's about *life*. And it's about making the most of that amazing woman you already are and believing in yourself to step into and claim your best and happiest life.

When you're trying to eat right, work out, and change your life for the healthier, it can seem like a lonely pursuit. But as we've come to realize over the years, people who are really successful at reaching their goals are those who feel like they have their very own cheering section. So as you begin your journey, principle by principle, know that we—and the thousands of others reading this book right now—are that cheering section. We may be writing to you in book format, but we are real people who live these principles each and every day. And, girlfriend, we—and all of the other FBG writers and readers on FitBottomedGirls.com—have your back. So just by picking up this book you have people all around the world who are doing this with you and cheering you on with fist pumps and corny you-can-do-it chants!

Change can be hard and scary, but don't let fear get in the way of becoming your best self. You aren't doing this on your own. You can always tap into the FBG online community by reading our daily posts and joining our conversations in the comments sections and on social media for instant pick-me-ups and motivation. So many women have become FBGs, and we're all ready to help you to become one, too!

The Fit Bottomed line? *You deserve to be the best version of yourself.* So join us on this journey to becoming a Fit Bottomed Girl!

CHAPTER 1

Ditch the Diet
(and Weight) Drama

Drama, drama, drama.

That's how we'd sum up the attitude that many women have when it comes to food, exercise, weight, and body image. It's like *The Young and the Restless* up in that headspace. But living a healthy lifestyle doesn't mean ricocheting among high highs, low lows, and badly acted plot twists. In fact, being a Fit Bottomed Girl is more like watching an episode of *Seinfeld* or *Friends*. You know what's going to happen, and you know you're just going to feel better because of it. Which is what this first principle is all about: *ditching the diet and weight drama, once and for all.*

"Diet"—as most people have come to understand it—is a four-letter word. It's about deprivation and torture and not having what you really want. It's about eating celery and carrots and going to the gym for hours *instead of* eating tasty food, spending hours on the couch watching movies starring Meg Ryan and Tom Hanks, and drinking copious amounts of wine (which, for the record, is how we spend many of our evenings and is a great use of a Friday night). This "diet" business is a drastic, unsustainable change in how you eat, with an end goal of reaching a number on the scale rather than achieving overall well-being. For many people, diet is about temporary results that lead to long-term dissatisfaction, guilt, and a sense of failure that chips away at not only your confidence to be healthy but also your overall sense of self-worth.

Like we said, drama, drama, drama ... .

Why Dieting Stinks

We probably don't have to tell you that yo-yo dieting stinks. But we will anyway, because it bears repeating. In fact, let us scream it from the proverbial rooftops: Dieting sucks! It blows! It's not a good way to live!

As we said, for many people the word *diet* is synonymous with deprivation. It means being "good." (Which, ahem, implies that you're "bad" the rest of the time?) Some diets feel like a torturous period you endure for as long as you can before going mad and being driven back into the warm and inviting arms of cheese, carbs, and chocolate. Some diets are about eating when you're "supposed to" and not eating when you're actually hungry. Many diets leave you saying no to the foods you love, totally ignoring your body's cues as to when and what you should eat. But if you're thinking about "going on a diet," doesn't that imply that you're going to eventually go "off" it? Whether you make it to the end of a specific program or give up beforehand, this attitude about dieting is not a permanent, healthy way of life.

There are too many ridiculous fad diets for us to list here—and anyway, we wouldn't want to give them the attention they don't deserve! But suffice it to say that most of these diets involve seriously restricting calories and/or food groups. And it's a given that they are not sustainable in the long term.

Why is it so hard to stay on a yo-yo diet for more than a week or two? First, your physiology plays a major role. Your body likes the status quo, and it wants to survive. And when you drastically cut the number of calories your body is used to getting, it thinks it's going to wither away and die. So all of these amazing and complicated processes start happening in your body, cranking your hunger levels way, way up. We won't bore you with the scientific specifics, but if you've ever heard of the hormones gherlin and leptin, they're at play here, making the odds of your long-term weight-loss success virtually impossible. Tricky little bastards.

You know that saying "Old habits die hard"? Well, it is true. While your motivation can power you through a crash diet for a week or two, in our experience it's just too much change all at once for any person to handle. Especially when you add in those aforementioned tricky little bastards causing you to want to eat your arm without sauce. Not only that, but when you are changing everything about how you eat and exercise at the same time, you have to spend a lot of time thinking about all of that. And that means a lot of brainpower goes to thinking about what you should—and probably what you shouldn't—be doing. As you undoubtedly know, human nature dictates that as soon as something is labeled "off-limits," we can't help but want that darn thing. Whatever the forbidden food is, it simply becomes incredibly irresistible—a giant pink elephant that you cannot stop thinking about. So instead of focusing on all the foods you *can* have, your brain becomes fixated on the ones you can't have, leaving you feeling deprived and miserable.

This is the reason many people don't keep their New Year's resolutions past January. Despite our best intentions and biggest aha moments, we are all creatures of habit. And while you can change your habits for the healthier, it's simply unrealistic to try to change all of them at once. That's why, as Fit Bottomed Girls, our goal is to tweak a little here, bit by bit, so that new habits are made and kept forever.

Crash and fad dieting have also been shown to do all kinds of other nasty stuff to factors other than your weight, such as weakening your immune system, harming your heart, and making you super cranky. (Okay, so there's no formal research on that last one, but we have had enough experience with it to know that being "hangry" is a real thing.) Extreme dieting has even been shown to reduce brain function, impair memory, and make someone more prone to depression. When you crash-diet, you're simply not giving your body the energy, vitamins, minerals, and nutrients it needs to function at its best!

Despite the fact that crash diets never work in the long term, we seem to all be obsessed with them. We all know people who have tried every fad diet out there, and they've "failed" at each and every one. But can we really call this "failure" when the fad diets don't work for anyone? Clearly, it's the culture of dieting that's broken, not you.

Which leads us to the reason we *really* discourage crash dieting: it drains your self-confidence. Because it is so hard to follow a crash diet for more than a few weeks, most people begin to think that they are personally to blame for not having the willpower to overcome their food demons. You think you can't do it. You think you'll never get healthy. You get beat down. And no matter how many different diets you try, the results are always the same. You lose some quick pounds, only to go back to your old ways, re-gain the weight, and feel that you'll never succeed. Every pound that creeps back on has chipped away at your self-confidence. This is no way to live.

How Not to "Diet"

In the next chapter, we give you some specifics of what and how to eat to really tune in to your hunger and listen to your body when it comes to cravings. But for now, we're asking you to make a vow to treat your body with respect. No matter what amazing results the next fad diet tries to sell you, remember that they're out to make a quick buck, not to give you the healthy lifestyle of your dreams. The short-term results you get from a fad diet are not worth the blow to your ego that will come when the pounds inevitably start sneaking back on.

Your body really does know what it's doing, and it will lead you down a healthy path—but you have to stop and listen to what it's telling you. Through years of extreme eating (that's what crash dieting really is!) we've spent so much time being told that we can't trust our instincts. But that's wrong. So instead of trying to make massive changes to your life and cutting out entire food groups, think about what foods give you energy. Pay attention to which foods bring you joy and which foods leave you wanting more. After eating a big ol' greasy pizza dinner, how do you feel? And how does that compare to the feeling you get after a meal of chicken, veggies, brown rice, and a piece of chocolate? What about when you hydrate with water instead of a diet soda?

Stop seeing foods as either "good" or "bad" and instead start really nurturing your body with food. While no foods should ever be totally off-limits, once you start to clue in to what foods make your body feel good, the decision of what to eat will become pretty darn easy. And be sure to check out the 10-Minute Fixes at the end of this chapter to help you to start listening to your body more attentively and to begin replacing junk food with simpler and more whole foods.

FROM THE FBGs
What We Wish We Could Go Back and Tell Our Younger, Non-FBG Selves

FROM JENN: It wasn't until before my wedding in 2007 that I "got" what living a healthy lifestyle was really about. In high school, I was active and worked out, sure, but did I do it for health? Eh, I did it more to fit in and be "skinny." It wasn't about how I felt or the energy I had—it was about looking a certain way. Or, really, *not* looking a certain way, as I definitely focused more on avoiding certain things (being fat) than on adding goodness to my life. By college, I was full-out obsessed with the number on the scale, the calories consumed, and how many hours I spent at the gym. I over-exercised, under-ate, yo-yoed, binged, drank too much, and was not being my own best friend.

That all changed before my wedding, though. I refused to walk down the aisle focused more on what I weighed than on what I was about to do: marry the love of my life. So I found a registered dietitian and I learned how to eat intuitively, listen to my hunger, and honor it (more on that in Chapter 2). I dropped my obsessions through lots of time and trial and error and unwavering self love (oh, how I wish this book was around then!), and I got on track. The process and difference inspired me so much that it became the inspiration for the mission of FBG. So what would I tell my younger self? Oh, plenty:

1. Any guy who thinks you'd be great if you just lost 10 pounds is never, ever worth your time. (And probably deserves a kick in the nuts.)

2. Use your time to study, laugh with friends, and be creative—not to add up calories or fat grams.

3. You are beautiful as you are, right this very second.

4. Cultivate friendships with those who bring out the best in your true nature.

5. Enjoy the journey. Everything is going to be A-okay.

You Are More Than the Number on the Scale

Who can relate to this scenario?

You wake up fresh in the morning and with tons of energy. You feel great. You've been working out, eating well, sleeping the right amount, and you are ready to tackle the day—no, you're ready to tackle the world! So you bound, naked as a jaybird (always weigh naked, right?), into the bathroom and hop on the scale. But . . . what's that? The number on the scale reads more than it did yesterday and even *last week*? But . . . but . . . You've been working so hard. How can it be? And then the destructive thinking starts: *I'll never be skinny. I can't do this. I'm destined to be overweight and unhealthy my whole life. I suck.* Head down, you get dressed in all black and have a terrible day.

Or how about this one: You've been eating healthy and working out regularly for a few days now, but then your boss comes in, drops a major last-minute project on your desk (sending you into a stress-filled panic), and before you know it you're in the break room eating donuts. Then you spend the rest of the day obsessively calculating how many calories you ate and what it'll take to burn them off. Later, you hit the gym and punish yourself with running, your least favorite way to work out but the only way you'll be able to burn the calories to make up for the donuts.

Now, looking at these two scenarios objectively, can you agree with us that it's crazy for your good mojo to be obliterated by a number that's flashing on some metal object you probably bought for less than $30? Should your confidence be shattered by a couple of dumb donuts? It's crazy. Instead of tying your self-confidence to things that really matter to your worth, like your character, your inner value hinges on how much you weigh or how many calories you eat. This means that one day you can be totally awesome and the next day totally suck. Not a great way to measure self-worth! Let's face it: there are going to be days when you snack on donuts instead of vegetables; there are going to be days when the scale tells you something you don't want to hear.

Never mind the fact that the number on the scale isn't even the best indicator of your health or progress. In fact, your weight can greatly swing—up to five pounds in just a day or two—based on simple things like hydration, sodium intake, or even if you've pooped lately. (TMI? No such thing in our—quite literally—book.) So if you're using the scale more than once a week to gauge your progress, you are not getting the most accurate picture of what's happening in your body.

You've probably heard about the body mass index (BMI), too. It's calculated based on your weight and height, but this number is too simplistic and—like the scale—doesn't take into consideration how much muscle versus fat you have on your body. In fact, based on the national guidelines of what a normal BMI is, many professional athletes are deemed overweight while many lower-weight and unfit people are called healthy.

And don't even get us started on those "ideal weight" charts that give a standard number for what men or women of a certain height should weigh. Really? With the diversity of bodies out there, we should all be a specific weight to be healthy? Sure, extra weight has its risks, but study after study has shown that you can have a few

ENERGIZE!
Pump up the Jams

Wish there were something to motivate you to exercise, to feel better while you're working out, and to keep your energy level up longer? There is, and it's no wonder drug. It's music! A 2008 study showed that people who listen to upbeat, high-energy tunes when they work out (Queen, Madonna . . . we bet your mind jumped straight to your favorite guilty-pleasure songs) can increase their endurance by 15 percent and generally feel more positive about their exercising experience.

The next time you need an energy boost, turn on some of your favorite high-energy tunes. If you're dragging at work around 3 P.M., pump up the jams rather than hitting the vending machine. And before your next workout session, put together a killer playlist. Try to pick songs that have a beat that can also act as a pacekeeper. You'll be amazed at how much the right song can keep you going—and keep you getting stronger!

extra pounds and still be fit and healthy. This is why we focus on measuring progress by other means.

So stop beating yourself up because of the number on the scale or obsessing about the calories you had at lunch. There is no magic number that will lead to eternal happiness, total fulfillment, and worry-free bathing-suit shopping. When you're living a truly healthy FBG lifestyle, you'll naturally settle into the right size for *your body*. You will look good, you will feel good, and you will be able to face any dressing room without fear. Promise.

Get a Cheering Section

You've likely heard the phrase "It takes a village" when it comes to raising kids. The same can be said for living a healthy lifestyle. Studies have shown that obesity can be "socially contagious," meaning that the habits and lifestyle choices of your friends can have a far-reaching effect on you. But the good news is that it also works for weight loss. Networks of supportive family and friends can play a role in your weight loss—and that's the reason commercial diets like Weight Watchers have meetings and support groups. Having a cheering section can make a lot of difference! Plus, it can make it tons more fun.

If you're at a loss as to where your cheering section may be, take a look around you. Maybe it's your partner, who is there for you through thick and thin (oh, we love our puns). Maybe it's your best friend, who is supportive no matter what. Maybe it's another family member whom you know you can go on a Fit Bottomed journey with or a co-worker who wants to avoid the unhealthy of-fice munchies, too. Look at the people in your life to find your cheering squad.

If you've taken inventory of all of the people in your life and still can't find that special support person, go online! That decades-old stigma of online relationships and friendships is gone, and there are now wonderful communities of supportive people just a few clicks away. Sites like SparkPeople.com and PEERtrainer.com are great for finding like-minded people. And we've also got daily doses of encouragement on FitBottomedGirls.com, so stop in frequently for encouragement and a sense of community. We'll also gladly take your emails with the success stories we know you'll have! No matter who is in your cheering section, check in often so that you can both give and get encouragement, and you can share your successes and stumbles.

FIT BOTTOMED MANTRA

"The past does not define you, the present does."
—JILLIAN MICHAELS

It's a Way of Life

You'll hear us say over and over that this book is about establishing a new kind of lifestyle, not going on a diet. We will hit you over the head with this point because we want you to really embrace this new mentality. Diets have start and stop points. But this is the best part of living the FBG lifestyle: *there is no destination and no end point.* This means that you can't fall off the wagon, even when you slip up! All of those typical diet no-nos? We're not going to tell you that you can't have them. Let there be chocolate. Let there be wine! We're going to help you find a way to enjoy what some diets might label as off-limits and also to enjoy the things that usually feel like burdens when you are dieting. (You might think we're crazy now, but by the time you reach the end of this book you are going to look forward to the times of day when you get to do some exercise!)

We think you'll find that once those foods aren't forbidden, they'll lose some of their appeal, and you'll enjoy them on occasion and in moderation, without ruining your progress. And guess what? When you're eating tons of foods that give you energy and make you feel awesome, you'll discover that some of your regular eats don't make you feel all that great anymore and you'll naturally stop craving them.

And did we mention that you can start living like an FBG only 10 minutes at a time? Read on, our little FBG in training, to put this principle in action. Ready . . . set . . . go!

So, we say to ditch the diet and weight drama, and we hope that this sounds like a good idea by now. But how do you actually do it, you ask? *For the love of all that is holy, HOW?!!!* First, have your inner drama queen stop using all caps and multiple exclamation points. Then, check out our 10-Minute Fixes. These quick fixes are designed to help you learn how to track your progress in ways other than stepping on the scale and to drop the diet mentality for good. They may seem simple, but once you start incorporating them into your lifestyle, they add up to a big difference in your Fit Bottom.

(1) BREAK UP WITH THE SCALE. If you find yourself hopping on the scale faithfully every morning—or worse, multiple times a day—it's time to break up with that scale. (We recommend weekly weigh-ins at most!) Take a minute to weigh yourself, then put the scale under the sink, throw it in your closet, or store it under the bed. Now, write yourself a note you can tape to the mirror that will tell you to turn away the next time you're tempted to dig your scale back out and weigh in. In the note, give yourself a short pep talk, and throw in a compliment or two, along with the reason you decided to kick the scale to the curb.

"Out of sight, out of mind" isn't working? If you need a momentary distraction to break the cycle, reach out to your support system to get your mind back on the positive. Pop onto Fit BottomedGirls.com—we hear they're always good for a healthy distraction over there. Once you break the scale cycle and move on to paying attention to other indicators of your well-being, you'll realize you're better off with just small doses of the scale.

(2) **MEASURE UP!** You know how people say muscle weighs more than fat? Well, that's not really true, as a pound of muscle actually does weigh the same as a pound of fat. What *is* true, though, is that a pound of muscle takes up four-fifths less space on the body than a pound of fat. This is enough of a difference to give two people of the same weight yet different body-fat compositions totally different clothing sizes! So as you get healthier and replace fat with muscle (check out Chapter 3 for specifics and workouts!), you'll measure key points on your body as a fab way to track that *sah-weet* progress. Just because the number on the scale doesn't budge, it doesn't mean you're not making real progress.

So rather than using that silly scale, get out a tape measure. It may seem old school, but it's a fantastic way to kick the obsessive "weighing yourself" habit, as well as to forgo the panic over day-to-day fluctuations. Tape measures are easily found in most sewing kits or at craft stores, and they are a simple yet effective way to really track your body as it adapts to a healthy lifestyle.

How to do it: This is easier to do with a buddy or loved one, but no worries—you can also do it as a party of one. Using a cloth tape measure, measure the fullest part of your chest, hips, thigh, and upper arm. Find your natural waistline—where your waist naturally curves in, not where your low-rise jeans hit you—and measure that, too. Make sure the tape measure isn't too tight or too loose, and keep it as level as possible. It's best to take your measurements *sans* clothes or in just your skivvies or swimsuit; just make sure to keep it consistent, whichever you choose. Most important: *Write it down so you can see your prog-*

ress over time! Over the weeks, you'll begin to notice some numbers going down (that's true weight loss), while a few might even go up a bit because you're building muscle (biceps, what what!).

We know it's tempting to bring out the tape measure weekly, but unlike the scale that fluctuates daily, inches take a bit longer to register. So, measure no more than every other week. Ideally, give yourself a month to see numbers that'll wow you. If after a month you haven't seen change, that's okay! Consider it a progress report and revisit the tweaks and changes you've made to your lifestyle to figure out what may not be working for you. Make sure you're following the FBG principles, and then hit up Chapter 6 about getting out of your comfort zone—it can do wonders for your progress.

(3) **SAY GOODBYE TO THE SKINNY JEANS.** Do you have a pair of skinny jeans that is taunting you? And we don't mean the skinny-leg jeans; we mean the pair that really hasn't fit you for two years but that you consider your gold standard for slim—the ones you try on to see if you've still got the ability to fit into them. Like measuring inches, fitting into a certain pair of pants can be a good indicator of progress. But—and this is a big *but*—if you find yourself stepping into them too often just to get frustrated that you can't zip them up, step away from them. Pack them away. Donate them. Put them in the back of your closet. They are driving you crazy, and FBGs do not let pants determine their success or failure!

Just as you're more than the number on the scale, you're also more than the size on the label of your skinny jeans. And your obsession with the pants? It may not even be about the pants themselves. Those pants likely take you right back to your glory days—to who you were, the fun you were having, the body you had. Don't let a relic from your past have that much power; you are awesome *now*. And your glory days? Look ahead for them, because they're coming at you.

Focus on the clothes that make you feel like a sexy beast. Your current clothes can actually be a great measure of your progress (as long as you're not only wearing maxi dresses and clothing with elastic stretchiness!). One easy way to track your progress is to see how your clothes are fitting. Do your jeans fit comfortably? Are they tighter than usual? Or looser? And how about that belt? Is it still in the same spot? Begin to be more conscious of how well your clothes fit, week after week.

So don't worry about those skinny jeans. If they're a pair of pants you truly love *and* they're still in style, keep them around. But like our recommendation for the tape measure, only step into them once a month. Remember: your new focus now is on being healthy and strong, not "skinny"!

(4) **PERFORM A CARDIO ASSESSMENT.** Remember the President's Fitness Challenge that you did in middle school? Well, after all this time, it's still a pretty good indicator of your fitness level, and it's a great way to track how quickly your body is adapting to the changes you're making. And don't worry; in our version, the cute boy you had a crush on won't be there watching your every move.

Testing your cardio fitness is as simple as doing a mile-long walk, run, or run/walk combination. Whichever you choose, simply truck it as fast as you can for a mile (four laps around a standard track). As soon as you cross the finish line, record your time. As your fitness level improves, you will see your times get faster. Mark your results down and repeat the test in a month to see how you've progressed. If you haven't improved as much as you'd like, don't fret. Just use it as an opportunity to set a new goal! Remember, being an FBG isn't about beating yourself up about what you can or cannot do, it's about loving yourself and your body for where it's at right now and then getting excited about what you can aspire to do in the future!

5 **TAKE A STRENGTH TEST.** Test your muscle strength with these basic moves that will act as a measuring stick for your muscle-building progress.

Crunch: Lie on your back with your knees bent, with the tips of your fingers touching your ears. Crunch so that your shoulder blades clear the floor, but don't do a full sit-up. Keep your hands lightly on the back of your head, but keep your chin lifted and focus on using your core—not your neck—to pull yourself up. Use a stopwatch to keep track of your time, and count how many crunches you can do in 60 seconds.

Push-up: For the push-up test, it's up to you whether you do a standard push-up or a modified one (where you're on your knees). Lower yourself with your elbows out wide so that you're about 2 inches from the ground and push back up. See how many you can do in 60 seconds.

Plank: The plank is one of those exercises that looks easy until you try it, but it's a move that will work your body head to toe, especially your core. Get in push-up position and then drop your elbows so that your forearms are resting on the ground;

your elbows should be under your shoulders with the rest of your body in a straight line. Time how long you can hold it. If you find this to be too difficult, drop to your knees and time how long you can hold it there.

Wall sit: Find your nearest sturdy wall, put your back up against it, and slide down until you are in a sitting position with your thighs parallel to the ground—like you're sitting in a chair without the chair. Using that stopwatch, see how long you can hold the wall sit and record your results. This is super challenging and really works the thighs and glutes.

Record all of your results and check back every few weeks to see how you're progressing. With regular workouts, you'll quickly improve!

(6) **TAKE A FLEXIBILITY AND BALANCE TEST.** Test your flexibility and how well you can balance with this quick test. Come on, get bendy!

Sit-and-reach stretch: Place a tape measure or yardstick on the ground, and mark off the 15-inch mark with tape. Place your heels at 14 inches (to account for your legs' movement as you stretch), with the 0 end of the stick toward your crotch. Touching the yardstick with your fingertips, reach out as far as you can and note how far you reached. Do this three times and record your best result.

Balance challenge: Simply try to stand on one foot for a minute. Now try the other foot. If those prove to be easy for you, try it with your eyes closed. Record your observations for each foot on a scale of 1 to 10, with 1 being the easiest thing you've ever done and 10 being climbing Mt. Everest.

As you start doing some of our workouts in the coming chapters, you'll see improvement in both your flexibility and your balance. Unlike strength, flexibility and balance are slightly harder to measure, but as your fitness level improves, you'll feel more stable and you'll notice that your muscles don't feel as tight as they once did as you stretch. Touching your toes won't be as difficult. You'll be a regular Gumby in no time!

(7) **CREATE YOUR HEALTHY SUPERHERO.** Ever wish you had superhero powers? Like the ability to turn down cupcakes? Or the power to run at lightning-fast speeds? For this 10-Minute Fix, we're going to help you harness those powers by creating what we call a "Superhero Alter Ego" who's a major healthy bad-ass.

For the next five or so minutes, brainstorm all of the fabulous characteristics of your Superhero Alter Ego. What can she do? What does she look like? What is she wearing? What's her theme song? (For the record, ours looks like Wonder Woman, rocks out to Gwen Stefani, and likes to curse.) Once you have her in your mind, either write down a description of her or draw her—nothing fancy; just enough to get the memory down pat. Then, when you're feeling a little off your healthy game or need a boost, think of her and act like her. Okay, you don't have to put on a cape, but play her theme song and embrace her healthy attitude!

Here's a fun thing about people: *we tend to value in others what we like most about ourselves.* So the Superhero Alter Ego you create in this 10-Minute Fix is actually, well, YOU! Cool, right? (We won't tell anyone that you like to be decked out in glitter and faux fur. . . .)

10-Minute Fixes

(8) RECLAIM THE SCALE. So you broke up with your scale. Hooray for you! But say you don't want to banish it to the landfill quite yet because you want to keep that once-a-week date with it. It's totally appropriate to check in with the scale once in a while, but you must follow the FBG commandment of not letting the scale mess with your mood. That's why we want you to take 10 minutes to reclaim the scale.

Make that date with the scale a happy time by decorating it—sticky notes with inspirational phrases, power words cut out of magazines, happy faces, puppies, whatever makes you smile. We want you to stick it to the scale. Phrases like "It's just a number" or "Perfect" or "Don't change a thing, dah-ling" can make light of any heavy associations you have with the scale. Having a "happy scale" can help remind you that, really, the number isn't the be-all, end-all, that the number doesn't tell the whole story, and that the number certainly shouldn't get you down.

(9) DECODE WHY YOU'RE IN THE DRAMA. So you say you don't like drama and that you want to break your obsession with the scale and with calorie counting, but you just can't seem to stop *thinking* about it? This is probably because of two reasons. First, our brains can get into ruts where we have habitual thoughts that repeat, almost without our realizing it. (Good news: By just being more aware and doing these 10-Minute Fixes, you can start to get your brain into healthier thought patterns!) Second, you might actually be *getting* something from the drama.

It may be that you need something to do with your time or that you like the attention of going on this diet or that program.

Maybe you view it as a way to feel that you have some control in your life. But the FBG lifestyle is a diet- and drama-free one, so take a few minutes to ask yourself this question: *Why do I like the diet drama?*

When you get an answer—no matter what it is—go a layer deeper by asking yourself: *Why do I need that in my life?* For a full five minutes, keep going deeper and deeper and asking "why?" and "why?" until you feel you have reached a real reason that resonates deeply. Then, spend the next five minutes brainstorming a few other ways to fulfill that need without obsessing about your weight.

We all have our reasons for doing things, even if we're not fully aware of them. But once you figure out *why* you're digging the drama, you can replace that behavior and dig yourself out of it and onto healthier and happier territory!

(10) **JOURNAL YOUR ANSWER:** *Why I'm more than the number on the scale.* For this exercise, write about why there is so much more to you than the number on the scale. What is that number not telling you—or someone who meets you? Why is a specific number important to you? What are your kick-ass characteristics that can't be measured by the scale? Don't worry about spelling or grammar; this is about letting your brain go and just writing. Set a timer for eight minutes and go!

Once you're done writing, go back and read what you wrote. Any aha moments? Learn anything new about yourself? Don't judge yourself as you read your answer; just learn and grow!

THE POWER OF THE PEN
Why Journaling Is an Essential Part of Your Journey

At the end of each chapter's 10-Minute Fixes, we've included a journaling exercise. Before you go rolling your eyes at yet *another* thing you have to squeeze into your busy life (we know, we know), hear us out. There is serious power in the journal—like change-your-life power, like Oprah-aha-moment power, like I-get-the-meaning-of-life-now power. Seriously.

We know it sounds over the top, but we've helped hundreds of others have huge, life-changing breakthroughs just by encouraging them to spend 10 minutes putting pen to paper. And research has shown that journaling reduces stress, improves mental health, and even can boost your immunity. Journaling regularly can also help you figure out what's been bugging you, help you to solve a problem, and even help you to know yourself better and uncover why you do (or don't do) certain things. Yes, it sounds a touch (okay, a lot) hippity-dippity, but it works. And it works especially well for finding your inner motivation, figuring out why you eat for reasons other than hunger, why you self-sabotage, and a whole slew of other, exciting self-realization prospects.

A lot of people avoid journaling because they think they have to be good writers. But the truth is that journaling isn't about writing, or spelling, or proper grammar at all. In fact, you don't even have to form complete sentences when you journal. Pick up a cheapo notebook at the store to noodle and doodle in, or write a note on your phone when you're waiting in line at the dreaded DMV. You can even write as a draft of an email or create an online diary, or use a computer's saved file for recording your thoughts. There's no right or wrong way to do it—just do it!

CHAPTER 2

Listen to Your Hunger

It seems like a no-brainer: eat when you're hungry and stop noshing when you're full. But somehow, over the years, something changed. We eat out of emotion (*We broke up; I need a pint of mint chocolate chip ice cream*), obligation (*But Grandma Millie made this special for me!*), and because food tastes oh-so-good (*Why is the combination of peanut butter and chocolate so darn irresistible?!*). We eat when we're "supposed to" and we don't listen to what our bodies are saying they really need. We eat on the go. We eat secretly. We starve ourselves. We stuff ourselves. Most of us have completely stopped paying attention to this basic bodily function!

No matter what kind of food you're eating (healthy or not!), when you listen to your *hunger*, we guarantee that you will begin to feel and look your best. When you retrain your brain to focus on eating when you're truly hungry and stopping when you're full, you will bring a healthy mindset to each and every meal you eat, setting yourself up for success over a lifetime.

So . . . who's hungry for more?

Eight Reasons Why We Eat When We're Not Hungry

In today's always-on-the-go, chaotic world, we eat for a lot of reasons other than just to quiet a growling stomach. Based on our own experiences and those of our readers, here are the eight most common reasons why we nibble when the hunger monster isn't actually calling.

1. **EMOTION.** We all have strong emotional ties to food. It's not a birthday party or wedding reception without cake. It's not Thanksgiving without turkey and pumpkin pie. Heck, can you even call baseball "baseball" without a beer and a hot dog? It's no wonder that we eat based on our heads and not our stomachs sometimes. We eat (and drink) to celebrate; we eat (and drink) to cheer ourselves up when we're down and out; we comfort ourselves with food and, in many ways, food becomes synonymous with love. So when we need love and support, we reach out to the safe arms of food (which never judge us, by the way—we usually handle that part ourselves, later).

2. **BOREDOM.** Sitting around? Got nothing to do? Why not eat?! It may seem silly when you say it like that, but a lot of us eat because we don't have anything else to do (or at least think we don't). And, yep, the food we pick usually isn't the healthiest of stuff.

3. **WE DESERVE IT.** What do a lot of us do after a long, hard day at the office? We hit happy hour and blow off steam with a cocktail and some fried foods with friends. And we don't just want the onion straws and cosmos; we have—in our minds, at least—earned them.

4. **WE *DON'T* DESERVE IT.** And "It" here could mean any number of things: the body of your dreams, the career you wish you had, the relationship you've been pining for. Basically, we eat to self-sabotage. It may seem counterintuitive (and in many ways it is), but sometimes we eat to punish ourselves or to keep ourselves from reaching our goals. We're convinced that we aren't good enough to succeed, and we prove ourselves right when we undermine our good intentions. No matter how many times you try to get healthy, if you're still thinking you're not good enough or that you don't deserve to live a fully healthy and energized life of your dreams, then you're likely to keep self-sabotaging.

FIT BOTTOMED MANTRA

"Our deepest fear is not that we are inadequate. Our deepest fear is that we are powerful beyond measure."

——MARIANNE WILLIAMSON

5. **IT'S THERE—AND IT TASTES GOOD.** Yep! Sometimes we eat—and can't stop eating—because it just tastes so darn good. And when we see food (especially the junk food), our brains get excited. In fact, one study found that when secretaries had access to candy on their desks, they reached into a clear candy bowl 71 percent more than into a white-colored one. Gives a whole new meaning to out-of-sight, out-of-mind, eh?

6. **PROCRASTINATION.** How many times have you found yourself looking into the fridge or perusing the goodies in the vending machine when you really should be doing something else? Yep, that would be

you, procrastinating. Usually we're using this delaying tactic because there's a stressor—whether conscious or not—that we're trying to avoid.

7. **OUT OF EXPECTATION.** This one is prevalent on birthdays, holidays, and, really, gatherings of any other kind as well. Someone made or bought food, and even though you're not hungry, you feel obligated to eat it. And so you do.

8. **WE'RE CREATURES OF HABIT.** Many of us learn early on to follow the "three square meals a day" rule, regardless of what our stomachs are saying. So it doesn't matter if you had a massive lunch; you eat dinner at 5 P.M. Or, on the other side of that coin, it doesn't matter if you are starving at 3 P.M. because you had a lighter-than-usual lunch; you eat dinner at 5 P.M. Overcoming some of these habits is as simple as being more mindful in your life (i.e., replacing unhealthy habits with healthy ones and learning how to say "Thanks, but no thanks" to foods at parties and such). However, other habits are a little more deeply rooted in our thoughts, feelings, and beliefs about ourselves, making them a little (okay, a lot) more challenging to fix. That's why eating according to your true hunger is such an important principle of becoming an FBG.

Healthy Eating Principles: Eat F-B-G

So you may be wondering: *Well, FBGs, what the heck do I eat when I am hungry? Does eating according to my hunger mean that I can eat anything, anytime I want it?* Good question, young grasshopper!

While we'd never, ever tell you to consider a food entirely off-limits. It clearly makes sense to eat healthy foods the majority of the time, with those yummy indulgences sprinkled in here and there. Remember how in Chapter 1 we told you to really start paying attention to how different foods make you feel? To consider how a piece of greasy pizza dragged down your energy levels one day versus some chicken and veggies another day? Well, that's what eating like an FBG is all about.

Almost like running your very own science experiment, start to play around and notice what foods make you feel good and what ones don't. Over time, you'll find that you won't think of these make-you-feel-good foods in the "healthy" way anymore—you'll consider them "normal," everyday eats! That is, when you're a full-fledged FBG, you won't have to force yourself to do or eat anything. You will enjoy what you're eating and it will make you feel good, so you *want* to eat it. No willpower required!

As you begin to see what foods give you energy and feel-goodness (yes, that's now a word) and which ones don't, we recommend you start with foods that meet the FBG criteria. They fit into a nice acronym, eh?

F is for Fresh. Yes, we're telling you to get *fresh*! But not in the feisty boudoir way; it's in the fresh food way! Fresh foods—aka whole foods like fruits, veggies, whole grains, nuts, seeds, and lean proteins—are chock-full of the good stuff that your body needs to feel its absolute best. These foods naturally boost your energy and fill you up.

So what about all that processed boxed stuff that's sold in the middle aisles of the grocery store—including the boxes of "diet" cookies and crackers? While they are convenient, it's best to stick to the whole foods that are found on the perimeter of the g-store.

In short, you want to mainly eat foods that have an expiration date—things that spoil and go bad after a week or two. (Sorry, but Twinkies and most other packaged "quick" foods don't fit the bill here.) Fill up on those "real" foods that have an ingredients list of items you can pronounce. Or, better yet, those that don't have an ingredients list at all!

B is for Balanced. Ideally, each meal and snack you enjoy should have a nice mix of carbs, protein, fiber, and healthy fat. Having a little bit of each ensures that your food is going to help keep your blood sugar levels stable and your belly full. The carbs give you energy, the protein helps build muscle and keeps you from feeling hungry, the fiber gets your digestive tract moving and grooving, and the healthy fat (think fresh like avocado, coconut, olives, and nuts) helps your body to better convert fat to energy and sends satiety signals to your brain.

We don't want to give hard guidelines on how many grams of this or percentages of that you should consume, because each day your body is going to need something a little bit different. So instead of obsessing about being perfect, just start to look at the makeup of your meals and snacks as a whole. Could you swap that sugary granola bar for one with more protein and fiber? How about adding a piece of avocado and some lettuce to your turkey sandwich? Maybe you could sub out those fries at dinner for a side salad with balsamic vinaigrette or a sweet potato?

Remember, it's all about balance, balance, balance!

G is for Gorgeous. No one likes to eat "diet" food, because it usually looks and tastes like cardboard. So choose foods that are appealing to you and take the time to create beautiful meals. Sit down at a table and eat off of a real plate, with real silverware. Ar-

SAY "SAYONARA, SODA"

We are huge proponents of eating, rather than drinking, our calories. It's one thing if your drink serves as a meal and is packed with tons of vitamins and nutrients (like a smoothie made with fruit, veggies, and yogurt). But it's quite another thing when it's packed with empty calories, as soda (pop) is.

Why is regular soda bad? Not only does it have *no* nutritional bang for your caloric buck, but it also has been associated with high blood pressure, a greater risk of obesity, increased risk of stroke, and even depression. But what if you're drinking zero-calorie diet soda? Well, you're not off the hook; some studies suggest that consumption of diet soda can lead to overeating simply because the brain expects those calories that didn't show up in the diet soda and later ramps up your appetite to get them.

Good old water is the best option for staying hydrated, so we recommend replacing a couple of your sodas with plain water or an unsweetened carbonated water each week. As time goes by, replace more and more of that soda with water so that you start thinking of soda as a treat rather than as a staple. For instance, maybe you'll only order soda on Fridays. Or you'll stop stocking it at home, but allow yourself to indulge when you dine out. Ideally, limit your soda fix to one serving a week. You'll probably find that you enjoy that one soda a week much more than when you were overdosing on it!

range the foods in a fun, creative, culinary-chef kind of way. Light some candles. Take a second before you eat to appreciate the food you're about to eat, and recognize just how lucky you are to eat something that's so good for you. And then slow down and enjoy each gorgeous bite.

Fresh . . . balanced . . . gorgeous. If the majority of your eats meet these three criteria, you're on your way to eating like an FBG! And if you need some ideas for how to turn these components into real, everyday meals, check out our Two-Week FBG Plan after the Additional Materials section at the back of the book!

Finding Portion Sizes That Are Just Right for You

Seeing that this chapter is all about honoring your hunger, you know that we have to talk about portion size, right? Because even if the majority of the food you're eating does meet our three healthy eating guidelines, that doesn't mean you should eat them with reckless abandon. In fact, the point of everything we're saying here is this: *begin to pay close attention to how much food it really takes to fill you up.* (And each person is a little different here, so don't base it on what your friends eat, especially if said friends are dudes.)

You don't need to measure everything to make sure your portion sizes are under control. Look no further than your hand for a general serving-size guide!

Fruits and veggies: size of your fist
Protein: size of your palm
Grains: half the size of your fist
Nuts: small palmful
Fats: size of your thumb

No matter what you're eating, you're going to feel better if you're not stuffed. We're sure ya'll have seen and heard the stats. Over the years, our food portions have gone from sane size to insane super-size, whether they are beverages or entrees, at home or served on restaurant plates. It is way too easy to eat too much almost everywhere you go. So we recommend acquainting yourself with portion sizes and being aware of how much you're really eating.

FROM THE FBGs
What Listening to Our Hunger Has Taught Us

FROM ERIN: I'm generally a happy, nice person. Until I get hungry. Those closest to me know better than to get between me and my next meal, lest they face the wrath of Hangry Erin—that's the Erin who's so hungry she's angry.

For years, I've been preventively avoiding Hangry Erin. Just a little hungry? Better grab a snack. Think I might get hungry in an hour? Might as well eat my meal now! I grew so afraid of turning into the Beast Who Must Be Fed that I realized I hadn't actually felt hungry in ages. When was the last time I actually felt hungry? When had I last let my stomach actually growl? And I couldn't remember. I had gotten so out of touch with my hunger cues that I was going through the motions, eating by the clock rather than by my true hunger.

So I started checking in with myself when I would instinctively head to the kitchen for a meal or a snack. Am I really hungry? Or did noon hit and I panicked because that's lunchtime? It took a while, but once I started letting myself get a little bit hungry, I realized that it wasn't the worst sensation in the world. I could survive Mild Hunger Erin.

Listening to my hunger has not only helped me avoid eating when I'm not even close to being hungry, but it has also allowed me to get in touch with my sense of fullness, so I can stop eating before I'm stuffed. Turns out, my stomach knows what I need more than the clock does.

Food and Mood: The Tricky, and Many Times Icky, Connection

Remember how "balance" is the second piece of eating like an FBG? Well, it's with really good reason, because when a food or snack is out of balance, it can have dramatic effects on your body. Addictive effects, even. Over the years, more and more research has shown that food addiction is a real thing. Certain combinations of food—primarily high fat, high sugar, and high salt—can be very addictive and can trigger reactions in the brain that are similar to those induced by drugs such as heroin and cocaine.

It seems that some people are more prone to food addiction than others, but we know that eating in a more balanced way (read: that nice mix of carbs, protein, healthy fat, and fiber!) is key to breaking the addictive properties of food. (As always, seek help from a professional for any serious psychological and disordered eating behaviors and issues.)

Using the Hunger and Fullness Scale

It may sound simple to eat when you're hungry and stop when you're full, but if you've been yo-yo dieting over the years, it can be a bit tricky, as many of us have learned to ignore the signs on both sides of the eating coin. That's why we recommend using a simple yet effective hunger and fullness scale to pay attention to your body's cues. It's amazing what your body will tell you when you're tuned in and listening!

On a simple scale of 1 to 10, check in with yourself about how hungry and how full you are before, during, and after each meal.

While it'll take some time and practice to figure out *exactly* how much food you need to fill you up and exactly how hungry you should be before eating, we recommend eating at about a 3 on the Hunger and Fullness Scale below and stopping when you're at a 7.

1   Starving! I will eat anything!

2   Can't stop thinking about how hungry I am.

3   Hungry, with an increased urge to eat.

4   A touch hungry. I could eat a little something, but don't feel like I have to.

5   Neutral. Not really hungry or full.

6   Not very hungry; feels like I still have some food in the stomach.

7   Hunger is gone. My belly is comfortably full.

8   Those last couple of bites were unnecessary. I've eaten plenty and I know it.

9   Starting to feel uncomfortable. Wish I had worn stretchy pants.

10 Thanksgiving Day full, plus. Uncomfortably and maybe painfully full.

Try taking a minute to do a thoughtful check-in before, during, and after meals to see where you are on the Hunger and Fullness Scale. You might be amazed at how different your eating habits will become simply because you're paying more attention to them! After a couple of days of working with the scale, you should start to get a good feeling for when to fuel up and when to put the fork down. Eating this way is not only better for your waistline but it will also help improve your digestion and give you more energy. You'll stop feeling bogged down by heavy meals, and as you learn to trust your body's signals, you'll begin to be more comfortable and confident around foods of all kinds—even the unhealthy ones—because you'll know that you can eat *just enough* to satisfy a craving!

In a Fit Bottomed nutshell, when you eat according to your hunger and choose balanced foods, you will simply set yourself up for a healthy lifestyle every time you sit down at the table to enjoy a meal!

If you've gotten out of touch with your body's hunger cues, or you find yourself eating for reasons other than true hunger too often, we're here to help. We promise that by tuning in to your hunger you'll be able to eat portions that are perfect for you and will enjoy healthy foods that will fill you and fuel you just right. Plus, here are some coping strategies for battling those emotional reasons you hit the cookie jar (or pickle jar or other jar of choice) and even some yummy food suggestions. If you've gotten into the habit of ignoring your body's cues, these 10-Minute Fixes will help you reestablish communication. We're practically a relationship counselor for your stomach-brain love connection!

1) **DISTRACT AND DELAY BEFORE YOU DISH UP.** It's amazing, but boredom is possible even when you're watching an enthralling reality TV marathon. Sometimes you just want something to *do*, and that something is to get up from the TV and go munch in the kitchen. So if you're feeling munchy but not sure that you're actually eating out of true hunger, distract yourself and do something productive—you know, those things on your to-do list that you just never get to.

For example:

- **Clean out your purse,** organize your junk drawer, or neaten your underwear drawer. You know they are total disasters.
- **Clean out your refrigerator.** That container with leftovers from two weeks ago? Taking a peak in there might make you lose your appetite.
- **Clean out your car.** We don't know how it gets that dusty, either.

- **Teach yourself to juggle.** (Lesson 1: Don't start with bowling balls.)

- **Get out of the house.** Sometimes you just need a change of scenery. Go for a walk around the block.

- **Call that friend** you never have a chance to talk to, or call up your support person and plan an active date.

- **Fit in a quickie.** We'll say no more.

- **Check in** on FitBottomedGirls.com and just try to limit yourself to 10 minutes. Ha!

Once your 10-minute distraction task is up, check back in with your hunger. If you're genuinely hungry, go grab that snack! If you've decided you're not hungry after all, you'll have an accomplishment under your belt and enjoy the satisfaction that you didn't just grab a bag of chips because you were bored.

(2) **VEG IT UP.** One FBG tried-and-true way to get more veggies into your diet is to take 10 minutes each Sunday to chop up veggies to use for snacks and salads all week. Throw carrots, celery, cucumbers, broccoli, cauliflower, bell peppers—you name it—into a large zippered plastic storage bag. Having the veggies already washed and chopped removes the energy barrier—they're ready to go!

(3) **TRACK YOUR INTAKE.** Nutrition labels on food packages are chock-full of information, but they're useful only if you know how to read them. You don't need to be a slave to the numbers, but knowledge is power when it comes to the items you use in the kitchen. For one day, collect the nutrition labels for the foods

you eat and write down everything you have eaten. Then take 10 minutes to add up all the great things your body gained— protein, fiber, vitamins, and nutrients—as well as the not-so-greats, like unhealthy fats and sugars. (You can also plug the items into free online food trackers, which will tally everything for you.)

When you're adding up your daily totals, remember to account for serving size; oftentimes, a package will contain more than one serving, so if you have more than what the nutrition label designates as a serving, you have to do the math to figure out your actual calories and nutrients.

Then take stock of your totals. Did you get enough protein? Do you need a little more fiber? Did one of your daily staples surprise you by its high sugar content? If your numbers don't look great, don't fret; knowledge is power! Now that you have a sense of how your everyday eats look, it will be a lot easier to figure out what you can tweak to make sure you're getting the best fuel for your body.

(4) **HYDRATE FOR THE DURATION.** Statement from Captains Obvious: Hydration is so important for your health. It helps your body run properly, from head to toe. But did you know that it can also help you in your weight-loss efforts? Yep! One study has shown that people who drank two cups of water before meals lost more weight than those who skipped the water.

Do you know if you're hydrated? We have an easy way to tell—in *way* less than even 10 minutes! Go pee. Yep—simply checking your pee is a good indication of your hydration level. It should be pale in color, like lemonade, not dark like apple juice. If it's not the right color, get thee to a drinking fountain or go refill your glass, stat!

You've likely heard the guideline of eight 8-ounce glasses of water a day. We say don't worry about hitting a specific target, but drink to quench your thirst and try to keep sipping all day long. And if you struggle with staying properly hydrated, set your phone's alarm every hour to remind you to take a couple of big gulps!

(5) **BE MINDFUL—WITH CHOCOLATE!** Now, here's a fun 10-Minute Fix: eat chocolate! But, wait, it's not exactly what you think! Okay, you do get to eat chocolate, but it's all about paying attention to the full chocolate experience. Which means that we're going to challenge you to take a whole *five minutes* to eat a small piece of dark chocolate.

Here's how it works: get a small piece or square of high-quality dark chocolate. (An individually wrapped piece of Dove Dark Chocolate works well for this.) Then unwrap it. Sit there with it in your hand and check in with yourself to see if any feelings start to emerge. Do you have a strong desire to eat it quickly? Do you feel anxious with it right there in front of you? Are you excited? Does your breathing change? What kind of thoughts are you having? Jot down your reactions on a piece of paper. Don't *judge* what emotions come up; just be aware of them.

Next, begin to look at the piece of chocolate. And we mean really look at it. Take note of the color and the shape. Feel how heavy or light it is in your hand. Look at it closely and then from farther away. Begin to notice how it smells. Is it sweet? Does it have notes of coffee or bitterness? Does it just smell really, really chocolaty? Get foodie with it, and note these reflections on your piece of paper, too.

Now the real fun begins! Set a timer (the one on your cell phone works great for this) for five minutes. Take the full time to really slow down and savor your piece of chocolate. Take little bites. Let them melt in your mouth. Experience the full flavor and mouth-feel of the chocolate. Let it rest on different parts of your tongue and see how the taste changes. Try not to think about calories or "if you're doing it right"—just slow down and enjoy the full experience of eating a piece of chocolate.

When your timer goes off, check in with yourself again to see if any emotions or feelings arise. Do you feel the need to have more chocolate? Or are you surprisingly satisfied with that small piece? Again, make a few notes on your experience, highlighting what you've learned from the exercise.

You can do this 10-Minute Fix with any food that you really, really love and that you crave. So, if you're more into salty and crunchy than sweet and melty, try this with a single potato chip or a french fry. The purpose here is to become more mindful when you eat. This exercise shows you that if you really slow down and pay attention, you can fulfill your needs with far less than you think. It's truly more about quality than quantity!

Also, if you feel some anxiety or have issues about food, this 10-Minute Fix will definitely bring them to light. For many of us, just having a high-calorie "treat" food around is enough to make us feel stressed or even obsessed—as in, *I need to eat that and I need to eat it NOW!* Until you tried this exercise, you might not have even been aware that you feel that way around certain foods. But the first step toward having a healthier relationship with food is becoming aware of what you're feeling and why that is so. In addition to being a fun way to satisfy your cravings in a healthy hunger-honored way, this little fix is also a bit of a window into your emotional-eating soul!

(6) **CHOOSE WELL WHEN THE ONLY OPTION IS FAST FOOD.** We know there will be times when you're on the go and your only option is the drive-thru. That's life! Sometimes you just don't have time to plan ahead. But instead of just pulling up and ordering that regular old no. 1 on the menu, you can research a few of the healthier options ahead of time. Take the next 10 minutes to browse the websites of the fast-food joints that you frequent the most—the ones you find yourself pulling into when you're short on time or making dinner just seems like too much effort. Taking the time now to find those healthier options will open your eyes to the fact that "fast food" doesn't have to mean a burger and jumbo fries.

Sure, fast-food options will never be the healthiest meals you can grab, but they don't have to be the worst, either. If a burger joint is your only option, order a regular burger *sans* cheese and go for a side other than fries, like apples, a cup of soup, or a side salad. The Subway chain has several 6-inch sub options that are under 300 calories—and you can load them up with lots of fresh veggies. Wendy's has a tasty low-cal chili (the large is only 310 calories, while the small one is 210). When opting for a fast-food salad, just be sure you watch the dressing and keep portion control in mind; some of the salad extras, like cheese, dried fruits, nuts (particularly sweetened nuts), and crunchy items like tortilla strips and croutons, can pack a massive caloric punch.

(7) **FIGURE OUT WHAT YOU'RE REALLY HUNGRY FOR.** Eating according to your hunger takes a little time and practice to master, which is why we offer this 10-Minute Fix: how to take stock of what you're really hungry for!

In that handy notebook of yours, do some food journaling with a little twist. Instead of just writing down your eats, also note where you are on the Hunger and Fullness Scale, both before and after eating. If you find yourself eating too much, or even eating too little (ending up too full or not full enough after a meal), throw a third question into the mix: *What am I really hungry for?* Ask yourself this little question before eating, take a deep breath to quiet yourself, and just listen to your body and mind. If you're physically hungry, a specific food like pizza or salad might come to mind. Or if you're not, something entirely different might pop up, like needing more energy, a break, or even some love or support.

Whatever the answer, meet it with acceptance and honor it. If your body really wants some roasted almonds and chocolate, have a little and savor every bite! And if you have an emotional need, meet it or make a plan to meet it soon, whether it's doing a few jumping jacks to give yourself a healthy perk-up, taking a 10-minute power nap, or dialing up a friend to chat. And believe

10-Minute Fixes

ENERGIZE!
Crank Up Your Vital Vitamins

A proper diet isn't just good for the waistline. Getting all of the right vitamins and minerals—and getting enough of all of them—is really important to feel your energetic best. Several vitamin deficiencies are linked to low energy levels, fatigue, and weakness, so boosting your iron, folic acid, and B_{12} might just boost your energy as well. Meat and lentils are good sources for iron, and B_{12} can be found in milk, eggs, meat, and poultry, along with fortified cereals. Folic acid can be found naturally in spinach, asparagus, and our favorite—avocado.

Your energy levels are just one more reason why it's so important to have a varied diet full of awesome foods; that way you can be sure you'll never be without a key piece of the energy puzzle!

us, it's simply amazing what your body will tell you when you're listening!

8 **DECIDE: IS IT HUNGER OR THIRST?** You've probably heard that sometimes you eat when you're thirsty rather than when you're hungry. You feel a need for *something,* so you head to the kitchen to grab a bite. But you've tried substituting a glass of water in this scenario and were left unfulfilled. Hydrated, but unfulfilled. So instead of just chugging the water, make hydration more of an experience.

Next time you're feeling a little hungry, take 10 minutes to make a special drink for yourself. Remember those cucumbers you sliced up, ready for you from 10-Minute Fix no. 2? Throw them into a glass of ice water for a refreshing drink with a spa feel. (Fruits and fresh herbs work in water, too, so experiment!)

You could also make a cup of tea; making tea is a soothing ritual in and of itself, and that's even before you sip it. Green tea, peppermint, chamomile, roobios, and oolong are all great choices. If after you take the 10 minutes to boil the water, steep the tea, and drink your cup, you're still hungry, by all means crunch away. But you'll know you're doing it out of true hunger. Win!

(9) **MAKE MEALS IN 10.** You don't have to spend a lot of time to eat healthy, filling, and satisfying meals. A few minutes of planning ahead before the week gets under way can set you up for later success. The following meal and snack ideas prove that not only can eating healthy be super fast but it's way more accessible than you probably thought—even if you've never been a fan of the kitchen (Erin readily admits to not loving to cook!). Our 10-minute ideas include all of those necessities in a meal that will make you feel satisfied—protein, fat, carbs, and fiber!

Bitchin' Breakfasts

Grab a bowl and go: Cereal is one of the fastest and easiest breakfast options, which is the reason there's an entire aisle at the grocery store dedicated to it. When you do eat it, make sure it's got the nutritional stats for stick-to-your-ribs staying power and won't just make you crash after a short-lived sugar high. Look for cereal with a few grams of fiber and fewer than 10 grams of sugar per serving. We love Rice Chex and Kashi Go Lean cereals for hitting these points reliably. Add a piece of fruit and some turkey bacon or hard-boiled eggs to your meal, and you're golden.

Sunrise sammie: You can actually make scrambled eggs in the microwave! Just whisk a few eggs, add a dash of milk (unsweetened soy, almond, or coconut milk work if you're not a fan of cow's milk), and throw it into the microwave for a couple of minutes. If you like, add some veggies like peppers, mushrooms, onions, or spinach to the egg mixture for an added nutritional bonus. Spread the eggs on top of an English muffin with a chicken sausage or veggie patty, and you've got a protein-packed sammie.

Not just for mares oats: Oatmeal is a filling, super-versatile morning meal that you can make in just a few minutes—and it can be different every day. Go for the basic, unflavored instant oatmeal so that you are the one in control of the sweetness and flavors. Then, for your toppings, get creative with fresh fruit, honey, granola, cinnamon and other spices, and nut butters like almond and cashew butter. Just be sure that you always have a little protein with your oats, be it a scoop of protein powder you've mixed in or a hard-boiled egg or two on the side!

Lickety-Split Lunches

Big-ass salads: Huge salads are staples around FBG headquarters. They're filling, oh-so-tasty, and tweakable until you find a combination you absolutely love. Check out our Big-Ass Salad recipe on page 286, too. Some of our favorite salad ingredients include cooked chicken (rotisserie or pre-cooked and sliced chicken makes it easy) or another protein source like chicken sausage, a salmon burger, or beans; chopped veggie mixes; and avocados, tomatoes, fruits, nuts, and cheese (feta or goat are yummy choices). Using pre-cooked and chopped items may add a little cost to your grocery bill, but the convenience, speed, and health benefits are huge!

Simple sandwiches: Just like our salads, there are a trillion sandwich options that yield fast, easy, and portable lunches. Some of our favorite sandwich ingredients are avocado, alfalfa sprouts, cucumbers, and peppers. Don't be afraid to add fruit, either; apple or pineapple slices can lend a sweet surprise to your sammie. You can mix and match meats—canned tuna, salmon, and nitrate-free deli meats are convenient options—and cheeses, and throw in different healthy bread options, like sandwich thins or pita bread for variety. As far as condiments go, add tons of flavor without tons of calories by using a tasty mustard (stone-ground mustard even adds a fun texture!), pesto, or even a flavorful hummus. You won't miss mayo one bit.

Din-Dins in 10

Shortcut soup: For quick soups, using a pre-made veggie soup as a starter is a great time-saver. One we love? Take a quart of a tomato or roasted red pepper soup, add nitrate-free pre-cooked chicken sausages, a couple handfuls of baby spinach, and a quick-cooking pasta like elbow macaroni or rotini. Once the pasta is al dente, you're ready to scoop and serve. Use this shortcut with other meats (cooked ground turkey is an easy addition to soups) for variety and for a way to throw in other veggies, like kale or chard.

Rockin' rotisserie chicken: Erin swears by the rotisserie chickens you can buy at the grocery store—they're affordable, versatile, and, hey! no cooking! Eat a chicken breast for dinner along with instant brown rice and a veggie or a mini Big-Ass Salad (*sans* the meat!). Use the leftover chicken for lunch salads or sandwiches all week long.

Snacks to Go in 10 Minutes, Alex

Nut butter mix-up: Apples, bananas, and celery have been paired with peanut butter since the dark ages. (We made that up, but it's a really long time, we're sure.) For a twist on this no-brainer, mix your nut butters—almond and cashew are tasty options—and fruits and veggies for endless possibilities. Carrots, jicama, pears, grapes, strawberries, peaches, cucumbers, and squash all make for a fresh take on the old favorite.

Fruit and cheese to please: Combine your favorite cheeses with a fruit for a protein-packed snack you'll look forward to. Top half a cup of cottage cheese with pineapple or another fruit you love, like berries. Grab a stick of string cheese and enjoy it with an apricot. Eat a Laughing Cow wedge with a handful of strawberries or a tangerine. Try an ounce of goat cheese with fresh cherries. You can't go wrong with any of these cheese-and-fruit combinations.

Yum hummus and veg: It takes just a few minutes to chop carrots, broccoli, and celery to dip in delicious hummus as a snack, and it's totally worth the effort. You can even buy mini carrots and bags of pre-chopped veggies to save time. Dip them in hummus as a go-to snack option that has a really nice blend of protein, fiber, and healthy fats. If you think you don't like hummus, try again: there are dozens of varieties and flavor combinations out there to taste-test. Just check out that ingredient list and look for the one that sounds the most natural.

(10) **JOURNAL YOUR ANSWER:** *How does food make me feel?* As with all of our journaling exercises, we don't want you to edit yourself or worry about spelling or punctuation. Just get down as

many thoughts on paper as you can in 10 minutes and write about how food makes you feel. How does it make you feel physically? What emotions do you associate with food? What foods do you love? Which do you hate? What meals make you feel fulfilled? What foods leave you unsatisfied? What are some of your earliest memories of food? What foods leave you feeling bloated and sleepy? Which foods leave you feeling perky and energized?

After your 10 minutes are up, review those notes and scribbles. Do you see any themes or emotions in your writing about food? Any lightbulbs going off in your brain? Learn from them and then move along!

CHAPTER 3

Move Your Body

We always say Fit Bottoms come in all shapes and sizes. But what's the one thing all of those fit bums have in common? They move—often! If you equate exercise with torture, it's simply because you haven't met the exercise equivalent of The One yet! You just can't be a Fit Bottomed Girl without the element of fun fitness. That's right—it's gotta be *fun* fitness. Because life is much too short to spend it slaving away on workouts you dread. We shall not stand for that!

First of all, there are so, so many exercise options available to you that you shouldn't waste any time doing something you don't love. From hiking, to Zumba, to lifting weights, to workout DVDs and channeling your inner Paula Abdul in your living room (that's not just us, right?), we'll get you moving and doing activities you truly enjoy. Plus, once you find workouts you love, you may be surprised at how quickly 10, 20, and even 60 minutes can fly by.

You don't have to commit to spending crazy amounts of time at the gym or hours each day exercising. While recommendations often call for at least 30 minutes of moderate exercise most days of the week, it's also beneficial to break those 30 minutes up throughout the day into more manageable chunks. And if you're just starting out, committing to 10 minutes can be a lot easier to manage than fitting in 30 minutes. Studies have even shown that exercise broken up into 10-minute sessions is more effective at lowering blood pressure than are 30-minute sessions. So if you're strapped for time, embrace a short workout session—your body will still get a lot of benefit from moving it for any length of time.

Besides gaining the health benefits of even small sweat sessions, fitting in short bouts of exercise during the day will get you into the habit of moving. As your fitness tour guides, we'll show you how easy—and dare we say fun?—it is to fit in your workouts. In our 10-Minute Fixes we've got workouts you can do at home, at work, even while watching TV. If you're a beginner, we'll get you moving for the first time. If you're a seasoned exerciser, we'll help boost your fitness levels. No matter what, we'll excuse-proof your workouts and help you learn to love the burn!

Ready to get moving?

Nine Reasons That Workouts Rock

We can tell you 'til the cows come home that exercise is amazingly awesome, but do you want a little more proof that regular workouts are the stuff that legends are made of? Well, we've got nine of those reasons right here. Giddy up, cowgirls!

1. **IMPROVES MOOD.** When you work out, your body pumps out feel-good chemicals called endorphins. These little guys give you that high-on-life, top-of-the-world, I-can-do-anything feeling and a general

sense that all is right in the world. In fact, exercise has such strong mood-boosting effects that studies have shown that it's good at preventing—and even treating—depression. Come on, get happy!

2.   **COMBATS CHRONIC DISEASE.** We know we said there was really no such thing as a "magic pill," but if exercise were a pill, it along with a healthy diet would pretty much be the answer to all of our chronic health issues. From cancer to diabetes, to arthritis, to heart disease, to asthma, and even back pain, exercise has been shown to help prevent or manage symptoms. Not to mention that people who move-it, move-it for about 30 minutes a day add another three-and-a-half years to their lives or even longer if they exercise at a higher intensity.

3.   **HELPS MANAGE YOUR WEIGHT.** We don't want you to get obsessive about how many calories workouts burn, but your body is made to move and burn off the energy (aka food) you eat every day. While today we live lives that are much more sedentary than our cave people ancestors, it only makes sense that getting active every day helps us to manage our energy balance and therefore keeps the pounds from creeping on.

4.   **BOOSTS YOUR ENERGY LEVEL.** Remember those feel-good endorphins we just talked about in no. 1? Besides improving mood, they also give you a better (and healthier!) boost in energy than any crazy can of high-performance, make-you-feel-like-a-bull-on-crack drink will. And the more you work out, the more efficient your heart, lungs, and muscles become. Over time, chores around the house and other physical tasks begin to feel easier—and you'll have more energy to do them so they won't take as long!

5. **PROMOTES BETTER SLEEP.** Getting your zzz's is super important for overall health and well-being, and studies show that regular exercise helps you to fall asleep faster, sleep longer, and have a better quality of sleep. And in our busy lives, who couldn't use a trick for better sleep?

6. **PUTS THE FIRE IN THE BEDROOM.** When you're fit, everything gets better, including the time spent underneath the covers. Active peeps tend to report having more sex and better sex—and active women may also find it easier to orgasm. From improved blood flow, to better body confidence, to the ability to get your body in creative and fun positions (yep, we went there), sex is an activity in and of itself and it's made better by sweat sessions outside of the sheets.

7. **MAKES YOU A SMARTY-PANTS.** When you're working out, you're not just training your muscles and heart, you're also training your noggin! Doing different exercises requires coordination and focus that challenge the brain, and may even help you to make new brain cells and establish new connections between brain cells that help you to learn. And if that weren't neato-bandito enough, even going for a stroll has been shown to fend off memory loss and keep skills like vocabulary retrieval large and in charge.

8. **BEATS STRESS (AND KEEPS YOU YOUNG).** There's no doubt that a workout can help you to burn off steam or anxiety. But researchers suspect that exercise may actually work on a cellular level to beat the effects of stress. In fact, researchers found that stressed-out ladies who worked out hard for an average of 45 minutes over a three-day

period had cells with fewer signs of aging than those who were pulling their hair out and were not active. So forget the beauty cream—hit the pavement!

9.   **CAN ACTUALLY BE FUN!** Um, hello! Working out is a really awesome way to spend half an hour (or more, if you want!) of your day. Life is short! The body is amazing! You are beautiful! Enjoy it!

FROM THE FBGs
Most Embarrassing Fitness Moment

FROM ERIN: Cardio Blast. The words sounded harmless enough. And so did the exercise class description: a "heart-pumping workout" using a combination of "athletic-based aerobic moves, step, Body Bars, hand weights, medicine balls and tubes" for a "high-energy" workout. I'm a high-energy kind of person; I'm in good shape. Totally manageable.

When I arrived to class, I first became concerned when I saw that everyone's steps were at the lowest height, no risers. Then I heard murmurs from the class. "Have you taken the beginner class? It's recommended before you take this one." Then I look around to see people *practicing their moves* on the step. What had I gotten myself into?

Up until that point in my life, I had taken one beginner-level step class, and it hadn't gone well. Slightly panicked, I looked at my options: leave the class with my tail between my legs before it even began or stay and get a workout and, likely, a laugh. Curiosity got the best of me, and I decided to stick it out.

I couldn't even keep up during the warm-up. For the entire 60-minute class, I wasn't in sync with the class a single time. Not once. The moves all had crazy names—Daisy! Bagel! Crab!

Batman!—and I didn't stand a chance. I bopped around on my step, laughing at the back of the room with another newbie who was in the same boat. It appeared that the other participants barely noticed us, because the moves were so intricate that even the well-practiced ones had to concentrate to stay with the pack.

By the end of the class, I was sweating bullets, most of which were from exertion and only a few from embarrassment. One participant commended us for sticking it out, and I was so proud of myself for not getting beat by a class simply because it was over my experience level. The instructor gave us high-fives and invited us to the beginner class. I took him up on it, and once those crazy step moves were broken down into manageable chunks, it became and remains one of my all-time favorite classes.

Get Started Putting the "Fit" in Fit Bottomed

Are you convinced yet that getting active isn't just a "must" but also an "OMG, I can't wait to do it!"? We thought so! So let's get down to the nitty-gritty on how to make getting active a "want-to" instead of a "have-to."

First things first: no matter where you are on your fitness journey, you want to incorporate the activities you love into your life. (Having trouble finding what these are? Check out this chapter's 10-Minute Fixes.) Remember, nothing is off-limits unless it involves sitting, so be sure to include every type of activity, from hiking to dancing to bad pop music, to playing with your dog or kids, to having raucous sex, to raking leaves and jumping in them. Make a point to do one of these activities for at least 30 minutes, three times a week. For beginners, this is the baseline amount of activity it takes to reap some of the awesome benefits we mentioned before and to also help get you into the habit of being active.

A lot of you might be hesitant to start getting active. You may have had negative experiences with exercise in the past or you may feel embarrassed just by the thought of putting on anything remotely resembling Spandex. And, ladies, we feel you! As a society, we've been conditioned over the years to believe that exercise has to be hard and torturous and miserable. But we've been thinking about it all the wrong way. Exercise in all forms should bring joy to your life—a means of celebrating and using your body in the ways it was intended. (Because as much as we like watching reality TV marathons, we're pretty sure we weren't created to do that . . .) So begin to see exercise as a way to live life more loudly, and step into the real you through it—the you who feels alive and good in her body!

Do not—we repeat, *do not*—allow your fear to stop you from doing the activities you love. If you're afraid to get off the couch because you think you might look like an idiot while doing that dance workout DVD in front of your husband and kids, take heart: no one can make you feel any certain way without your permission. So no matter what activity you want to do, do it with a whole lot of self-love. Stay focused on why you're getting active.

And if you're totally, 100 percent clueless about what activity to start with, we recommend walking. It's free and there's no learning curve. And even if the weather sucks, you can still march in place inside. No excuses! Start wherever you can, however you can. The first step is always the hardest, but with every step you take, it gets easier. And more fun. We promise.

The point is to move and make it a regular part of your day that

ENERGIZE!
Simple Tricks to Get Pumped for a Workout

The toughest part of doing a workout is taking the first step. It's simple physics: bodies in motion tend to stay in motion; bodies at rest tend to stay at rest. So if you're having a hard time with those first few steps, here are some tried-and-true tricks!

Get dressed. You can't have a proper workout without dressing for it. And sometimes throwing on a super-cute workout outfit is all you need to remind you of why you want to hit the gym.

Promise 10 minutes. Pretty much everyone can do pretty much anything for just 10 minutes. Even you! So commit to it and then plan something you're looking forward to. (Hint: Check out our 10-Minute Fixes for a workout you can fit into your day!) Take that first step—whether it's putting in that DVD, getting out the front door, or going to the gym. Once you do the first hardest step, you'll feel silly not finishing the workout!

Musica! You know that song that is your anthem? That gets your hips swaying and has you channeling your best pop diva whenever you hear it? Yes, that song. Throw it on. The beat just might be enough to get you moving! Studies have shown that exercisers increase mileage and heart rate with faster-paced songs. Even though you might not feel that the workout is easier, you'll enjoy it more with your favorite tunes.

Mantra mania. Whether you borrow from Nike's slogan "Just do it," find inspiration from one of the mantras sprinkled throughout this book, or make up your own saying, repeat your mantra to yourself to get yourself revved up and ready to go!

you look forward to. It's not something you dread or always want to skip. Once being active switches in your brain from a "have to" to an "I get to," the FBG magic happens. You no longer have to "force" yourself to work out; you just want to do it and so you do! And day after day, "doing it" leads you to make being active just another normal part of your everyday life. Getting to this fitness Promised Land might take weeks or months, but that is totally normal and okay. In fact, it's good because you're building a true *habit* of living a healthy lifestyle and not just on one of those dreaded "plans" you start and then stop after a short while. And we promise that once you make being active a habit, you'll look back and wonder why it took you so long to get started.

Now, for those of you who are already active, doing the things you love, and are looking to take things up a notch, we've got plenty of info for you to get you to the next level, so just hang tight. And for you beginners, again, just focus on getting into the habit of being active. Once there, you'll soon be ready to spice things up and push yourself a little harder, which, of course, we have suggestions for doing in our 10-Minute Fixes.

The FBG Fitness Triangle

Now, once you've gotten the hang of being active, and you've made it more of a no-brainer habit (like buckling your seat belt or brushing your teeth), you may want to take it to the next level. So let us introduce the FBG Fitness Triangle. A triad of cardio, strength, and flexibility, this is an ideal mix of workouts that together deliver true full-body fitness and whole-body feel-goodness. (And don't worry; we've got a sample Two-Week FBG Plan at the end of the book for you to see how this gets put into exercise action.) While any activity is good, this combination is an ideal way to work out once you've already made the habit of being active and are loving it. And there are plenty of ways to customize the triad so that it works for you and is something you really enjoy.

Think of "fitness" as a triangle. And on each point of the triangle, there's an important piece of the fitness puzzle. While each piece is awesome on its own, they're most awesome when they all come together—as they will give you not only a rockin' body (bonus!) but also a strong heart, healthy lungs, the ability to do everyday tasks easily, and the greater likelihood of preventing injury. Basically, you'll feel a hell of a lot better physically and be able to do all the things you want to do!

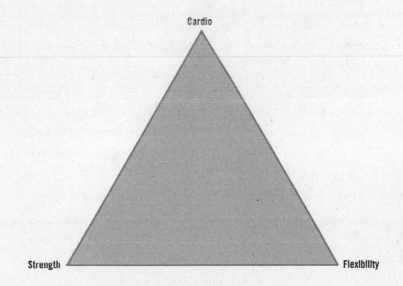

You've probably heard these three words thrown around—cardio, strength, flexibility—but here's why they're so important and why we recommend you do activities each week that hit all of them to make up the full FBG Fitness Triangle.

Cardio: Aerobic exercise or cardiovascular exercise is what most of us think of when we think *exercise*. It's the stuff that gets your heart pumping and makes you sweat. It's anything that gets you out of breath—by a little bit or a lot—including walking, running, dancing, jumping, hiking, and skiing.

Your heart is basically a big muscle, and when you move enough to get your heart rate up above a resting rate (you know, the one that the doc records each time you visit?), you work it. And the more you work it, the stronger it gets. Regular cardio exercise has been shown to decrease cholesterol levels, improve heart function, and reduce the risk of heart disease—even reduce the risk of osteoporosis.

Strength: The second point in the FBG Fitness Triangle is good ol' strength. Somewhere along the line we ladies got it into our heads that weight lifting and muscle building were just for the boys, but that couldn't be further from the truth. Strength training is insanely important to our overall health, body composition, and metabolism. In fact, because lifting weights does have a slight cardiovascular component to it (when you lift something heavy you get out of breath, right?), it has most of the benefits of cardio plus it helps to maintain your muscle mass as you get older, which then helps to prevent weight gain and reduce your risk of injury.

Flexibility: Whether you consider yourself flexible or not, working on your "bendiness" is a major tenet of good fitness. Regular stretching can reduce the risk of injury, allow for a greater freedom of movement, reduce stress, and just make you feel more graceful and beautiful.

For some reason, a lot of people hate stretching because they

WHERE DO YOGA AND PILATES FIT IN?

The great thing about both yoga and Pilates is that they combine flexibility work with strength training. They're full-body practices that work you from head to toe and are awesome at hitting your core—all those muscles in your trunk and pelvis that help stabilize you in your everyday activities. They also make great active recovery workouts and are perfect for days when you want to get in some exercise but you don't want to do your regular cardio session. Both practices focus on body positioning and proper alignment and the breath, and as such require lots of mental focus. Being more mindful while you exercise can also help you tune in to your body, your emotions, and even your hunger when you're out of the Pilates and yoga studio. These types of workouts can range from relaxing to vigorous, so play around with classes and types until you find something you love!

feel that they're not good at it. But in order to get the benefits, you don't have to be a master yogini, or even be able to touch your toes! Stretching a little bit most days of the week or doing some yoga poses and respecting your body's natural limitations is enough to see improvement and get those healthy goodies we mentioned above.

When you put these three tenets together, you get one heck of a fit and well-rounded FBG!

The Ideal FBG Workout Plan

By now you're probably asking yourself: *Self, how does one do all of this in a week of workouts?* And, if so, your self would be asking a wickedly good question. Here's our answer: the Ideal FBG Workout Plan. It all begins with a base of nutrition, hydration, and rest days.

Good nutrition: To properly support your workout regimen, you must get the proper nutrition to fuel your workouts. You want your legs to be shaky from working them to fatigue, not because you didn't eat properly before your workout. Not getting enough food can be counterproductive—instead of the pounds dropping off, your body will actually hold on to extra weight no matter how many miles you log on the treadmill.

Want to eat for your best workout? Follow these guidelines!

- *1–2 hours before a workout:* Eat a small snack that has some carbs and protein and not a lot of fiber. Also, make sure it's a food your belly tolerates well! We like half a peanut-butter sandwich or half of a banana with a tablespoon of almond butter.

- *During your workout:* As long as your workout isn't more than 90 minutes, water should be A-okay! If it is longer than 90 minutes, you'll want a sports drink or an energy gel.

- *After your workout:* The sooner the better, but definitely within an hour after exercise, get some protein and carbs in yo' belly! About 10 to 20 grams of protein seems to be best for muscle recovery. We suggest trying a protein smoothie with fruit, a few slices of nitrate-free deli turkey with an apple, or cottage cheese with chopped raw veggies.

Proper hydration: If you want to stay alive, drink water. Obviously. But beyond survival, maintaining hydration is essential for good athletic performance. Dehydration leads to muscle fatigue, loss of coordination, and muscle cramping. Your body also loses its ability to cool down properly and won't have the energy it needs. None of these conditions makes for the best workout, right? So drink up before, during, and after your workout to give your body the hydration it needs, whether you're just taking a walk or going for an hour-long run.

Rest days: Just as you need proper nutrition to fuel your workouts, you also need rest. To properly build muscle, those muscles actually need time to repair and rebuild. Working out too much will just make you fatigued and probably cranky. Plus, rest days are crucial to prevent overuse injuries and mental burnout. Rest days aren't a license to totally veg out, though—you can have active recovery days with an easy yoga DVD or a walk in the park. You just want to make sure you're not hitting up the same muscle groups day after day, with no rest. Ideally, you want to skip a day after working a specific muscle group. And if you're super sore after a workout, take a day or two off before you hit those muscles up again.

Now that you're well fed, hydrated, and know that rest is super-duper important, let's get to putting those three fitness tenets—cardio, strength, and flexibility—into action. Workout action! Yes, we know it looks a little intimidating, but we swear it's actually quite simple. The idea here is to get maximum awesomeness in short amounts of time, so always pick activities that you enjoy!

1. **STEADY ROCKING CARDIO:** *2–3 times a week, 10–60 minutes.* This workout only requires that you do something that you love and that gets your heart rate up for at least 10 minutes at a time—run for 10 minutes or jump on the elliptical for 30 minutes, or go to an

hour-long class of booty-shaking Zumba. It doesn't need to be crazy hard—just enough to get you a little out of breath but not so out of breath that you can't talk.

2. **HIIT IT:** *1–2 times a week, 10–30 minutes.* Hold on to your fit butts! HIIT stands for High Intensity Interval Training. Now, you may already be familiar with interval training, in which you alternate levels of a harder intensity with an easier intensity—for example, running for a minute and then walking for minute. But HIIT is like that, *plus.* Instead of just working a little bit harder during your intervals of a higher intensity, you work a *lot* harder. Like as hard as you can. So instead of a run/walk workout, you do a sprint/jog or sprint/walk workout where you push yourself so hard that you are totally out of breath and can only get a word or two out. And then you recover—to do it again!

You can do HIIT with both cardio-based workouts, like the running ones we mentioned, or you can do them with strength-based moves, like kettlebells swings or jumping lunges. HIIT doesn't require a certain amount of time for the intervals, so you can kind of have fun with the times, but we prefer that the high-intensity part doesn't last more than a minute or two without some kind of recovery to get your heart rate back down to a more moderate level where you can speak a little bit.

Interval workouts are incredibly effective at boosting your overall fitness because they push your cardiovascular system so much. But because they're so taxing, your body also needs lots of rest from them—hence our recommendation to do them just one to two times a week for 30 minutes or less!

3. **GET STRONG.** *2-3 times a week, 10-60 minutes.* Through either body-weight training (push-ups and sit-ups) or by lifting actual weights like dumbbells, bars, or even bags of flour at home, you want to challenge your muscles to get stronger. As you build muscle, you'll burn more calories, improve your cardio endurance (stronger muscles

WHY CIRCUIT STRENGTH TRAINING ROCKS (AND SAVES YOU TIME!)

What happens if, in a pinch, you just can't fit in all of the components of the FBG Fitness Triangle in a week? Or you can squeeze in a few workouts but not meet the requirements of the ideal workout plan? No worries! Besides cutting yourself a break (hey, life happens!), the secret to staying fit when life gets crazy is multitasking. And in the fitness world, *multitasking* means "circuit training." With strength circuit training you can do double duty with your workout by getting strength and cardio in *at the same time*. End with a few stretches and boom! The FBG Fitness Triangle is met.

So what exactly is circuit strength training? It's an interval-based way of working out whereby you do one strength move and then push on to the next move without rest in between. Because of the fast-paced, no-rest nature of circuit training, it's not an easy workout, but it goes by quickly because you're doing so many things back to back.

The sky is the limit on how many moves you do, what moves you perform, and how long your circuit lasts—so it's also a workout that beats boredom. (For specific ideas to get you started, be sure to hit up the 10-Minute Fixes at the end of the chapter.) Not to mention that circuit training is also a form of HIIT, meaning that you burn tons of calories in a short amount of time, boost fitness, and may even pump up your metabolism with a 48-hour post-workout afterburn effect. Talk about short-circuiting your way to fit success!

mean cardio becomes easier), and improve your body composition (less junk and more muscle in the trunk!).

Don't worry about bulking up: unless you plan to lift ridiculously heavy weights for four-plus hours a day, eat only protein, *and* take performance-enhancing drugs, you will not find yourself looking like a bodybuilder. Our goal is to give you a toned and strong body that reflects your inner strength. And remember how we told you that muscle takes up less space on the body than fat? Well, strength-training workouts are how you change that body composition to have more muscle than fat!

4. **GET BENDY:** *5–7 times a week, 5–10 minutes.* At the end of every workout, or even while watching TV or before going to bed, take just a few minutes to stretch. It doesn't have to be anything fancy—just a couple of leg, chest, back, and arm stretches or even a few yoga poses will do it. But take a few minutes to improve your range of motion, limber up, and de-stress. If you do a lot of workout DVDs or go to group exercise classes, most will include a little stretching at the end of your workout just for this purpose. And if you regularly do yoga or Pilates, go ahead and count that as getting bendy!

Just because we're giving you "a plan" doesn't mean that ya'll can fall into the trap of all-or-nothing thinking or perfectionism. We know that life happens, so use this as a *guideline*. And as we keep saying again and again (broken record, right here!), play around with what feels good for you and your body. We find this mix of workouts to work well for most people and get great results, but everyone is a little different. So listen to that body, do what you need to do, and find the fun!

Whether you're new to the exercise scene or a seasoned workout pro, these 10-Minute Fixes will introduce you to new—and fun!—ways of fitting in workouts and falling in love with the sweatier side of life. With so many awesome options, you'll be well on your way to making a habit of fitness and having it be part of your everyday and totally awesome life because you want to, not because you feel like you "have" to!

1. **FIND YOUR PERFECT WORKOUT.** You've read this whole chapter and still can't think of anything that you like to do that could be considered active? Take a couple minutes to jot down on paper your honest answers (your first reaction is usually the most true one) to the following questions. Some of them may seem out of left field, but they have a purpose. (We always have a method to our madness!)

- What kinds of activities did you enjoy doing as a kid?
- Think of the last time you felt good and alive in your own skin What were you doing?
- Are there any activities you've always wanted to try but haven't?
- When you go on vacation, are there active things you enjoy doing?
- What's your favorite type of music?

   Now, go back and review your answers. Were there any com mon elements? Say you loved playing soccer as a kid and the last time you felt good was when you were playing in your work softball tourney. (You may want to consider signing up for an adult team sports league!) Or, you have always wanted to go skydiving and love going on hiking trips. (You love being in nature, so you should try running and walking outside.) Or you love high-energy dance tunes and feel you're best on the dance floor. (Zumba or Jazzercise might be the best thing to ever happen to you.)

Really think about the activities that bring you joy and choose workouts that echo those elements. If you're a social butterfly, try a group ex class with friends. If you love being quiet and being meditative, seek out a yoga DVD. The only "perfect" workout is the one that you do regularly—and love!

(2) **FIND A GYM FOR YOU.** Health clubs can be intimidating. (You're not dreaming—much of the equipment does, in fact, look like torture devices.) But, if you can find the right place, gyms can be a healthy refuge. They can be a place you go to focus on you and your healthy living goals, a place to fall in love with new workouts and have a good time. But how do you find a fitness center that's right for you? Carve out a 10-minute block and then do the following:

- Call a few of your friends who belong to health clubs. Ask where they go, why, and if they'd recommend it to someone like you. We've found that word of mouth is the best way to get real, honest feedback on a place.

- Hop on the Internet and look up the health clubs in your area. Do you like the services they offer? The tone of their writing? Does the overall feel of their website pump you up? Or does it give you visions of lunkheads grunting and slamming down weights? Do they have generally good reviews? Are they female-friendly? You want to be open to all possibilities, but go with your gut here.

- Narrow it down to one or two clubs to try. From there, call them and schedule a time to visit that's at the time you'd be most likely to go.

When you do visit a gym, don't feel pressured to join, but do make sure you feel great about the place. Check out all of the facilities and even chat with other members to see if they'd recommend it! Keep looking until you find a perfect fit.

(3) **TRY THESE CARDIO, STRENGTH, AND FLEXIBILITY PLANS.**
As we discussed earlier, the ideal FBG workout plan incorporates cardio, strength, and flexibility training. So no matter where your exercise is taking place, we ask that you pick some moves from each of those categories and integrate them into your day. You can do them all in a row or break them up, but incorporating a little bit of each type of movement into every day will get you results that you won't believe. Here are some suggestions.

CARDIO WORKOUTS

Are you a cardio queen? Or aspire to be? Try one of these fun and easy steady-state cardio workouts, or even do five minutes of two of them for a mix-and-match quick cardio burst! And want to make it a HIIT cardio party? Simply up the intensity for a minute with the following HIIT options, and then recover for a minute. Repeat five times and you're done!

Cardio Workout 1: Dance to your favorite tunes. Pop on some good tunes and get moving and grooving for three or four songs!

HIIT option: Really exaggerate those dance moves with high-impact and full-body dance moves like the Running Man or doing the MC Hammer shuffle. Recover with easy dancing.

10-Minute Fixes

Cardio Workout 2: Walk, jog, or run outdoors. Lace up your
sneakers, get outside, and take a couple of laps around the
neighborhood!

HIIT option: If you're walking, jog to up the intensity. If you're
jogging, take it to a run. And if you're running? All out sprint it,
baby. Recover with a slow walk.

Cardio Workout 3: At the gym. Get on a piece of cardio
equipment that has a form of resistance, like the elliptical,
stair-stepper, or bike, and start moving!

HIIT option: Crank up the resistance so that it takes all your energy
and focus to get through the movement. Recover by lowering
the resistance down to easy peasy.

STRENGTH WORKOUTS

We said strength workouts work, and believe us, if you do these
strength workouts regularly, you will definitely see yourself get
stronger!

Strength Workout 1: Short circuit. Grab a set of weights—
5 pounds to 12 pounds each—or even something heavy in
your house that you can hold, like cans of food, jugs of water,
or even a cast-iron skillet (those suckers are heavy!). Then
do 20 reps of the following moves. See how many times you
can get through this circuit in 10 minutes, or as much time
as you have!

- **Shoulder presses**
- **Lunges**

- Bicops curls
- Squats
- Sit-ups with your feet resting underneath the dumbbells' handles

Strength Workout 2: Deck of cards. This is a really, really fun one! Take a shuffled deck of cards and randomly pick a card. The number indicates how many reps you're doing of a move (face cards equal 11, aces equal 1). Then match the suit to the following moves:

♠Crunches

Be sure not to use your hands and momentum to crunch yourself up. Focus on using your abs to slowly bring your shoulder blades off the floor, keeping your eyeballs up and on the ceiling and your chin off your chest.

♦Push-ups

Whether you decide to do these on your toes or on your knees, keep your body as straight as you can as you lower down and push back up. Don't let that booty drop down or pop up!

♥Lunges

To better ensure proper form, step backward to do your lunges, coming down so that your front leg is at 90 degrees and then pushing back up. Oh, and when you get your number, left/right equals one. Gotta keep it even on each side!

♣Squats

We like doing these over an actual chair and then touching our booty to the seat to make sure we're really dropping down and are keeping our knees behind our toes as we lower. And for an added bonus, give your booty a squeeze on the way up!

Do 25 mountain climbers

Start your mountain climbers in a plank position, with your whole body straight. Keep your abs in as you drive your knees into your chest. If you're a newbie, get your knees as close to your armpits as you can. If you're an advanced exerciser, try to get your feet to and even past your armpits. Ah, yeah.

Get through as many cards as you can in 10 minutes, and if you have more time, try to get through the full deck for a *killer* workout. And, of course, feel free to adapt this general idea to your favorite moves. Just about anything will work, from burpees to triceps dips, to high knees, to jumping jacks—so have fun crafting your own special "deck of cards" workout!

Strength Workout 3: Five minutes to the burn. This is a two-part workout. The first will work your legs; the second works your upper body. Get ready for it!

First five minutes: With weights on the ground and in your hands, do a push-up (either on your knees or on your toes). Hold plank for 30 seconds. Do another push-up. Still in plank position, row the right weight up, pulling your shoulder blades together, and then place back down on the ground. Repeat on the left side. Come out of plank/push-up position. Rest for 30 seconds. Repeat the whole thing again as many times as you can in five minutes.

Second five minutes: Get down in squat position like there's an imaginary chair behind you, with your knees not going over your toes. Hold for 30 seconds. Stand up and then lunge forward on your left and then your right. Stand back up, lower down into a squat, and jump up twice. Rest for 30 seconds in standing position. Same drill as the first five minutes—repeat the whole thing again as many times as you can in five minutes.

FLEXIBILITY WORKOUTS

Ready to get bendy? Try one of these three workouts to stretch and lengthen your bod!

Flexibility Workout 1: Basic stretch series. Whether it's at the end of a workout or at the end of a long day, this basic stretching sequence is just delightful. It'll leave you and your muscles feeling oh so good.

- **Body openers,** 60 seconds: Take deep breaths as you lift your arms overhead and back down. Breathe in as you raise your arms up, and breathe out as you lower them back down to your sides.
- **Easy neck rolls,** 30 seconds: Slowly circle your head each direction, bringing your ear as close to your shoulder as is comfortable.
- **Back stretch,** 30 seconds: Interlace your fingers and bring them in front of your body, rounding your back and feeling a stretch between your shoulder blades.
- **Chest stretch,** 30 seconds: Interlace your fingers and bring them behind your body, pushing your chest forward.

- **Biceps stretch,** 30 seconds: Take your arms out to the side, pushing your thumbs down and away from you, feeling a stretching throughout your arm.

- **Standing forward bend,** 30 seconds: Lean forward until you feel a mild point of tension. Hang there, with a slight bend in the knees.

- **Quad stretch,** 30 seconds each side: From a standing position, have your left hand grab your left foot behind you. Keeping your knee pointed down, bring your heel toward your rear until you feel a stretch in the front of your leg. Repeat on the other side.

- **Calf stretch,** 30 seconds on each side: From a standing position, push your left leg back behind you, keeping your knee straight. Drive your back heel onto the ground, feeling a stretch in your calf. Repeat on the other side.

- **Hip flexor stretch,** 30 seconds on each side: From a standing position, push your left leg back behind you, bending your knee so that you're in a lunge position. Hold that lunge while you drive your hips forward so that you feel a stretch in your hip flexor. Repeat on the other side.

- **Butterfly stretch,** 30 seconds: From a seated position, put the bottoms of your feet together in front of you with your knees bent and to the side. Bring your feet closer to your body until you feel a stretch in your inner thighs.

- **Butterfly reach,** 30 seconds: From your butterfly stretch, fold your torso down and over your legs to deepen the stretch.

- **Side bend,** 30 seconds each side: From a seated position, extend your legs as far apart as is comfortable. Sitting tall, reach out and over to the left side, keeping your chest lifted and tall. Hold there as you feel a stretch in your opposite side and your leg. Repeat on the other side.

- **Twist,** 30 seconds each side: From a seated position, extend your legs and take your left leg over your right. Sitting tall, twist to the left and hold. Repeat on the other side.
- **Give yourself a hug,** 30 seconds: Thank yourself for taking care of you today! Smile! Feel good!

Flexibility Workout 2: Zen it out. Yoga is a fabulous way to stretch and quiet the mind—and even sneak in some muscle building! Do these slowly, being sure to breathe deeply and fully through each movement. Hold poses for 20 to 30 seconds. Do the series as many times as you can in 10 minutes. You should be able to get through it a few times, but focus more on stretching your body and flowing with the movements rather than focusing on how many times you can get through the series. Slow down and enjoy it!

- Stand tall (mountain pose)
- Deep inhale up, reaching arms up and overhead (upward salute)
- Swan-dive and fold your upper body over (standing forward bend)
- Take your leg back and into a lunge (alternate legs each time you go through the series)
- Come into plank
- Open into side plank on the left side (alternate sides each time you go through the series), return to plank
- With your arms close to your side, lower down to the ground (either from your knees or your toes)

- Lift your upper body slightly off the ground into upward-facing dog
- Push your hips up and back into downward-facing dog
- Walk your hands back up to your feet so you're back to mountain pose

Flexibility Workout 3: Roll out. Truth time: we have a love-hate relationship with our foam roller. Basically just a cylinder of dense Styrofoam, you probably have seen these at your gym, as they are fabulous for loosening up tight muscles and preventing injury. Problem is—similar to how a deep-tissue massage is awesomely good for the muscles yet doesn't exactly *feel* relaxing—foam rolling can be a bit intense, too. However, if you're someone who sits for hours on end, runs a lot, or tends to have hip, knee, or back pain, a roller can do wonders for the body.

You can pretty much "roll" any muscle on your body, including your quads, hamstrings, IT band (which runs on the side of your leg and is notoriously tight in runners), hip flexors, back, rear, and calves. No matter where you roll, though, the main thing you want to do is to slowly roll over a muscle, using your body weight as pressure. When you feel a spot of tightness or straight-up ouchiness, hold there for about 30 seconds, breathing deeply. Doing this helps to loosen tight muscles, break down tiny knots, and generally make your muscles more smooth and able to move in a better, more natural range of motion.

Spend some time playing around with the foam roller and seeing what muscles on your body are tight, and then focus there. We won't lie: sometimes you will find a spot that hurts, big-time. When you do, feel free to adjust your body weight a little so that you aren't putting as much pressure on the tight spot. A little pain is okay with foam rolling, but if you're ready to cry and scream uncle, you may need to back off a bit. And that's okay, as you can build up to it over time. In fact, the more regular you are about your foam rolling, the easier and less painful it becomes.

And, dudettes, there is no better feeling than when you stand up after a 10-minute foam-rolling session. It's like your entire body has been reset to how it's supposed to feel—longer, stronger, and more relaxed. It's like magic for lengthening tight or overused muscles. And it's the one time you'll ever hear us agree with the motto: no pain, no gain!

(4) TRY AT-HOME WORKOUTS. Home may be where the heart is, but it's also where a fantastic workout can be, too. Here are three ways to get your sweat on at home sweet home!

At-Home Workout 1: One-minute home circuit. This is a full-body strength workout that does not disappoint. Do one minute of each of the following moves, except where noted, in this order for a strength-and-cardio-in-one workout that doesn't require any equipment except a chair and some energy!

- **March in place to warm up: 30 seconds**
- **Push-ups**
- **Mountain climbers**
- **Triceps dips off of a chair**
- **Backward lunges**

- Burpees
- Squats
- Jumping jacks
- Crunches
- Plank hold
- March in place to cool down: 30 seconds

At-Home Workout 2: Jumping stairs. If you have a jump rope and the space to do it, go for it. If not, just use your imagination and jump up and down like you do have one.

0–1 minute: Step up and step down on a stair
1–2 minutes: Jump rope in place
2–3 minutes: Do push-ups with your hands on the stair
3–4 minutes: Jump rope in place
4–5 minutes: Put your right foot up on the stair; lunge down and up
5–6 minutes: Jump rope in place
6–7 minutes: Put your left foot up on the stair; lunge down and up
7–8 minutes: Jump rope in place
8–9 minutes: Do triceps dips on the stair
9–10 minutes: Jump rope in place

At-Home Workout 3: Tabata. Looking for an at-home HIIT option? Tabata would be it. Based on the Tabata Protocol, which has been used (and gotten amazing results!) in exercise science research, it's simply doing a move all out for 20 seconds, followed by just 10 seconds of rest, a total of eight times. In 10 minutes, you have enough time to conquer two moves, plus a minute for a warm up and a minute for a cool down. And believe us, this is so intense that you'll need it!

For Tabata, grab a timer and choose one move from each category below. Although you can do both strength or both cardio, we like doing one of each to get the best of both worlds!

STRENGTH MOVES

- Push-ups
- Triceps dips
- Lunges or jumping lunges
- Squats or squat jumps
- Plank or side planks (alternate sides for each 20-second interval)
- Crunches or full sit-ups

CARDIO MOVES

- Mountain climbers
- Burpees
- High knees
- Jump rope
- Jumping jacks
- Skater lunges
- Stairs
- Jogging in place

Warm up with a minute of walking in place, do your two eight-round intervals of Tabata (each round should take you four minutes, in case you lose count!), and then cool down with a minute of deep breathing and easy stretching. Whew. You did it!

FIT BOTTOMED MANTRA

"Do the work. Do the analysis. But feel your run. Feel your race. Feel the joy that is running."

—KARA GOUCHER

(5) DO TV WORKOUTS. TV time is prime time for zoning out and relaxing. But if you struggle to find time to work out, TV time can also be the perfect opportunity for exercise. These two TV workouts will have you moving no matter what you're watching!

TV Workout 1: Reality TV. Reality television is nothing if not predictable. But that predictability lends itself to some serious workout potential. Use this guide like a drinking game, only this is way healthier! Each time the below scenario happens, do the matching move.

Someone cries: Do 10 jumping jacks
Someone is bleeped: Do 10 squats
Someone is under the influence of alcohol: Do 10 lunges
Someone says "thrown under the bus": Do 10 push-ups
Someone says "it is what it is": Do 10 triceps dips
There is a physical altercation: Do 20 mountain climbers (10 on each side)
Someone walks off camera: Hold a plank as long as you can
Someone gets kicked off: Do a wall sit for as long as you can

During commercials, add in cardio elements—interpretive dance to match commercials, marching in place, faux jump rope, kickboxing punches. Pick a movement and keep your body going. Depending on the show you're watching, you could get one heck of a workout before an hour's up!

TV Workout 2: Sports sweat. If you're a rabid sports fan or live with one, odds are good that the TV is tuned to games for hours on end. And those hours could be used for some killer multitasking and muscle building. Think you'll feel silly? Make your viewing partner participate. If both of you are doing it, it'll be twice the fun! You could do these for just 10 minutes or you may find it so fun that you keep doing them for the game's duration. It's up to you!

Basketball

Free throws: During free throws, alternate faux jump shots with marching in place for plenty of cardio in a foul-heavy game.

Time-outs: Alternate these moves during time-outs: squats, lunges, push-ups, and planks.

Technical foul: Do 15 burpees.

Football

Your team scores: Do a push-up for the total number of points. So the first time a touchdown with an extra point is scored? Do seven push-ups. The next? 14. And so on. The higher the score, the buffer your arms. (Feel free to mix it up with triceps dips!)

A flag is thrown: Do a cardio element for two minutes.

Jumping jacks, walking in place, high knees, your hottest dance moves. Mix it up so you don't get bored.

Time-outs: Have dumbbells nearby for biceps curls, overhead presses, triceps kickbacks, side raises.

Baseball

Hits: Whenever someone hits the ball, run laps around the room (or in place) while the batter runs the bases.

Home run: Run in place while the runner runs the bases, and at each base, jump as high as you can and reach for the sky. At first base, jump once. Second base, twice. Third, thrice. Home, four times.

Each out: Alternate 10 each: mountain climbers, lunges, squats, calf raises, push-ups, leg lifts, and crunches.

Walk: If a batter walks, hold a plank as long as you can.

Stolen base: If a runner steals a base or attempts to, do lateral jumps as wide as you can for one minute.

Huddle at the mound: Faux jump rope for the duration of the pitcher pep talk.

No matter what you're watching, use TV as an opportunity to get off the couch—and not just to veg!

6 **CHOOSE AN AT-WORK WORKOUT.** It's entirely possible to get a workout in while you're at work. This workout is ideal if you've got an office door and can close the door for 10 minutes (perfect if you're bored to death on a conference call!). But if you're in cubicle land, we'll help you sneak it in around the office. (Because healthy living is great, but you might not want to appear totally crazy doing push-ups in the hallway, right?)

Walking cardio: Do a 2-minute walking warm-up. Either head outside for a quick walk around the block or do a quick lap around the perimeter of the office indoors. Head to your car to grab something you "forgot" to get a quick breath of fresh air. Taking a file or stack of papers with you can make this endeavor look totally legit.

Stairs: Hit the stairs for 2 minutes. See how many flights you can cover and then head back down to your floor. If you don't have stairs, tack two extra minutes on to your walk.

Bathroom business: The bathroom isn't just for doing your business! Head to the privacy of a stall to get in some squats by lowering yourself into a seated position and hovering just above the toilet. Do this for a minute. The next minute, use the stall door to do 20 push-ups at an angle.

Ab power: You can work your abs all day every day, but sometimes you need some reminding. Isometric ab moves—where you hold your stomach muscles tight—can work your abs without anyone ever knowing it. Sitting at your desk, simply tighten the muscles of your abs and core. Think of squeezing your entire midsection in as tight as it can go. Visualize bringing your belly button to your spine while you bring your pelvic floor muscles up and in (Kegels, anyone?). Hold each contraction for 20 seconds, rest for a couple of seconds, and repeat for 2 minutes.

Leg lifts: Seated leg lifts strengthen not only your quads but the muscles surrounding your knees, plus they stretch your hamstrings while you're at it. In a chair, sit up tall, keeping your abs in, with your feet comfortably resting on the ground. Then straighten your leg, tightening your quads and the muscles around your knees. Hold for 5 seconds and repeat on the other side. Alternate sides for 2 minutes.

Seated side stretch: Sitting up straight, reach one hand to the sky. Stretch to the side as far as is comfortable to stretch your obliques; hold for 10 seconds. Alternate sides to cool down for a minute. Bonus if you roll your ankles at the same time.

(7) CLEAN IT UP. Cleaning the house is already an active endeavor, but there are ways to pump up the jam when it comes to making it a workout. You'll feel the burn and see the sparkle with each of these quick exercises you can add to your clean routine.

Tub scrub and lift: While you're already down on your hands and knees scrubbing the bathtub, add some butt toning to the mix. Stretch your leg out behind you and do 10 leg lifts on each side before you rinse the tub.

Vacuum circuit: Vacuuming the floor is guaranteed to work those guns, but make sure you're alternating arms to get the benefit on both sides. Each time you enter a new room, do 20 lunges before continuing to sweep.

Laundry squats: Have a load of laundry to fold? Place the basket on the floor and squat deeply each time you have to grab a new piece of clothing to fold.

Dust race: Make the dreaded dusting chore a little more active and fun by setting a stopwatch and dusting a room as quickly as you can. Next time? Try to beat your time. Bonus: you get it over with as quickly as humanly possible.

Backyard burn: For outdoor chores you don't even have to add any extra moves to get a workout. Mowing the lawn with a push mower? Cardio and strength city. Raking leaves? Great arm workout. Trimming bushes? Your guns will be smoking.

Weeding the garden? Full body toning. Washing the car? More full body toning. Just focus on doing these quickly and with vigor, and they can totally count as exercise!

8) **MAKE A WORKOUT BUCKET LIST.** Variety is the spice of life, and trying new workouts will keep your workout life fresh. Plus, you never know when you'll find that new workout routine that you adore. To help you stay excited about workouts, take 10 minutes to find new workouts and fit adventures you want to try. Is there a hiking trail you'd like to check out? A new workout trend you've heard of and meant to look into? An exercise class only offered in Italy?

Take to the Internet and research options both near and far. One great place to get inspiration? Search Pinterest for "fitness." Dream big and forget limitations of locale and expense. Want to hike the Grand Canyon? Try white-water rafting? Go rock-climbing? Learn to play tennis? Take that Bollywood workout class? If you've thought it, put it on that list! When you put the ideas out there, you'll start looking for ways to make them a reality. Make it a goal to mark one off this year and take a first step in the direction of that dream. If it helps, recruit a workout buddy or fit friend to make it happen.

9) **GET FAMILIAR WITH YOUR HEART RATE.** Your heart rate is a great way to measure your fit progress, and it's also a fabulous indicator of how hard you're working when you're exercising. The fitter your heart is, the fewer the beats it takes to pump your blood through your bod. Take 10 minutes to check in with your ticker!

Find your resting heart rate: Check your pulse when you've been resting for at least 10 minutes—first thing in the morning is the perfect time for this. Find your pulse—your wrist and neck are easy options—and grab a stopwatch or a watch with a secondhand and count your pulse for 30 seconds. Multiply that number by 2 for your resting heart rate. A normal heart rate for adults ranges from 60 to 100 beats per minute (bpm). Super-fit athletes have heart rates in the range of 40 to 60 bpm, so the lower the rate, the better. Write down your resting heart rate and check it again after a couple of weeks. It's great proof that the workouts you're doing are really benefiting your heart!

Find your target heart rate: Your target heart rate is where you want your heart rate to be when you're working out. For moderate intensity, the target heart rate should be 50 to 70 percent of your maximum heart rate. For vigorous exercise, the range is 70 to 85 percent of your maximum heart rate. Do a little math to find your zone. Subtract your age from 220 (your maximum heart rate) and multiply by the percentage. This example is for a 30-year-old.

50%: 220 − 30 years old = 190 x .5 = 95 bpm
70%: 220 − 30 years old = 190 x .7 = 133 bpm

So for a 30-year-old working at a moderate intensity, the heart rate should be between 95 and 133 bpm. Vigorous intensity for this same person would be between 133 bpm and 161 bpm.

Now, these numbers are helpful, and if you have a heart rate monitor, that's the easiest way to check in throughout your work-

An Easy Way to See How
Hard You're Working

Just as you don't need to be a slave to the scale or to calorie counts, you don't need to be a slave to your heart rate numbers all the time! That's where the "rate of perceived exertion" (RPE) comes in.

RPE Scale

0–1   No exertion at all: Lying down.

2–3   Light exertion: Walking.

4–5   Medium exertion: Brisk walk/light jog. You're feeling warm.

6–7   Moderate exertion: Think running. It's getting tough to hold a conversation.

8–9   Hard exertion: Think sprinting. You can't say more than a couple of words at a time.

10   Maximum exertion: Think sprinting up a hill, with weights. No way you can talk.

Use the RPE scale to check in with yourself as you exercise to see how hard you're pushing yourself. Aim for somewhere between 4 and 7 for a moderate-intensity workout. When you're doing HIIT workouts, your intervals should hit an RPE of 8 to 9 and your recoveries can be more in the 4 to 5 range. And if HIIT seems *too* intense, try doing a more moderate-intensity interval workout by working at a 6 to 7 and recovering with a 3 to 4.

out to see if you're working hard enough. If you don't, though, you can simply take your heart rate for 15 seconds while working out and then multiply that number by 4 for your bpm.

(10) JOURNAL YOUR RESPONSE: *How amazing my body is.* For this exercise, spend 10 minutes reflecting on and celebrating your body and all of the amazing things it can do. Even if you haven't reached your goals yet or are frustrated that push-ups still feel *so darn hard*, take this time to really appreciate your bod and celebrate your achievements. What can your body do that has surprised you? What can you do now that you couldn't do before? How are your muscles changing? Anything you take for granted? How do you feel when you eke out that last push-up? What would you like to try? Once you're done writing, reflect back on how awesome and strong your body is—and remind yourself to carry that appreciation into your daily life.

CHAPTER 4

Take a Balanced Approach—to Everything

It's so easy to let your life get off balance. It happens before you realize it. Obligations pile up, work deadlines loom, friends and family demand your time and attention. Before you know it, you're stressed and feeling frazzled and worn out. It's never fun feeling stretched too thin, as if you're burning the candle at both ends, with work, family obligations, friend drama, romance, and working out. But balance isn't just a buzzword we want you to incorporate into your diet and exercise. Balance is a lovely philosophy for your overall life!

You've probably heard the saying "All good things in moderation." Heck, it's a catchphrase on FBG, we say it so much! But it's not just a cliché. Well, it *is* a bit of a cliché, but it's one that is so meaningful and important. All good things in moderation—which will henceforth be known as AGTIM (catchy, huh?)—is a phrase that FBGs live by because it helps us be balanced in *all* areas of our lives. From your workouts, to your food choices, to your career, to your family, to your relationships, and anything else in your life, AGTIM helps you to maintain a sense of wholeness and complete well-being. After all, when one area of your life is out of whack, it tends to put other areas of your life off-kilter, too. You've probably seen that in your own life when work gets too crazy or a family member gets sick and needs extra care. We bet you've thought about it wistfully, when you've decided to go on some crazy crash diet and can't eat anything but grapefruit and tuna. We know for sure that you remember it after you've worked out too hard or too fast and have gotten injured.

When things are out of balance—and you ignore your intuition to slow down, powering through from this thing to that without enough downtime—you just don't feel your best or have lots of energy. You feel stressed, anxious, irritable, tired, and down: pretty much all the things that being an FBG *isn't* about.

We'll be the first to admit that "finding balance" is a bit elusive. Being balanced isn't something that you can do or not do; it's more of a flowing and continuous process that is built on the choices you make every day, if not every minute. But being more balanced is possible, and over the course of this chapter, we're going to take you through what you need to know so that you can feel fabulously balanced more often!

What Does Balance Mean, Really?

As we said, balance is a bit difficult to really "find" and keep hold of. One day everything might feel like it's humming along and all key areas of your life are equally being attended to, and the next— well, you might get a flat tire, have to work late on a big project,

FROM THE FBGs
What Balance Is

FROM JENN: When I feel balance in my life—a sense of being in control and aware of everything and also in a really good positive and happy headspace—it's like nothing can stop me. When I'm out of balance, though, things just have a tendency to feel . . . off. There's not enough time to do the things I want—and need—to do, and I just don't feel as passionate or motivated as I'd like.

Over the years, though, I have gotten better at finding balance and keeping it. Writing about healthy living is my passion, but sometimes I don't know when to hit the pause button. I've approached burnout—and gotten there—quite a few times. So much so, that writing an email felt like torture. And those dust bunnies under the couch? They'll bring a girl to tears.

That's why, for me, balance is a constant process of checking in with myself and working little mini-breaks into my daily routine so that I don't push myself too hard. Multiple times a day, I stop what I'm doing and check in with myself. I see how I'm feeling. I go walk the dog. I meditate for 15 minutes. I never eat at my desk. And I try to read at least a few lines from an inspirational book every day to keep my noggin grateful and focused on the good in life. (And, seriously, there is so much good in life!) Doing this helps me to better balance my day. It ensures that by the time 6 P.M. rolls around on a Friday, I have the energy and desire to be more than a cranky bump on a log.

I know that being 100 percent balanced all the time isn't realistic. Life happens! But by making an active effort to think about the important aspects of my life that I want to have in balance, I'm able to keep my priorities where I want them and not spend too much time worrying if one day calls for more attention in one area than in others. And when I'm balanced, I'm happy!

and then come home to a sick kid. And poof! Balance gone. On the opposite side of that, when you're on vacation, sitting on the beach and drinking a mai tai, you might feel as though you are perfectly balanced, that life is as it should be. But we guarantee that if you did that, and only that, for a month, you'd soon feel bored, sluggish, and notice that your clothes aren't fitting as nicely as you'd like them to.

So what is balance, really? Balance is *not* about having a perfect day or being happy 100 percent of the time. It *is* about living real life with a healthy attitude and positive habits. In FBG land, balance is making sure that all your core needs are being met. You're eating healthy foods that give you the fuel you need. You're moving your whole body in ways you love that give you more energy. You're going out and being social, but you're still sleeping enough. You're enjoying a glass of wine with dinner, but not four glasses of wine with dinner. You're working toward your goals without making too many sacrifices in the rest of your life. You know how to say no—and yes. And, of course, you treat yourself with love and compassion.

Being balanced is a constant give-and-take; you have to be flexible and fluid about your plans and your life. It's the push and the shove, and the yin and the yang. And finding the just-right mix is a little different for everyone. That's why we're here to help you find it!

Balancing Your Eats

So what does moderation mean when it comes to your eats, and how does that translate into your daily life? To us, moderation in our diet means that nothing is off-limits, but that we make it a point to have the best, healthiest foods most of the time. As you work through this book and you start hearing what your body is saying to you, you'll start to notice the foods that leave you feeling awesome. The ones that don't upset your stomach. The ones that don't leave you feeling sluggish. The ones that satisfy you and don't give you a sugar high—and crash. The ones that wake your body up. These are the foods you want to focus on, the ones you want to make up the bulk of your diet. (Was that a fiber joke? We think so!)

To live "moderation" in your diet, try thinking of it as an 80/20 split. The majority of your choices—the 80 percent—are healthy ones, like fresh fruits and veggies, whole grains, healthy fat, and lean proteins. That leaves 20 percent for the fun splurges, like alcohol or dessert or a slice of your very favorite pizza.

Sure, some days and weeks may look more like 75/25. Other days the split may be more 90/10. But make 80/20 your goal, and you'll find that it's a great balance of healthy awesomeness and fun. See our quick fix later in this chapter (page 114) to check in with yourself to make sure you're really living the 80/20 principle.

Balancing Your Workouts

You know that working out is awesome. And in Chapter 3 we went over the three elements of the FBG Fitness Triangle, so you know that ideally you need a balanced approach to fitness that includes cardio, strength training, and flexibility work. We know that it can seem like a lot to fit in three different types of workouts, especially if you're still caught up in a little of the dieting mindset where you *always* want to burn as many calories as possible. After all, some of the workouts we recommend, like yoga, Pilates, and stretching, don't even get you sweaty! But remember, being an FBG isn't about working out to your hardest every day. It's about the slow and steady increase in fitness that you can do—and enjoy—for a lifetime of FBGdom! So what does this ideal mix of workouts look like in terms of a normal week? Again, it's about all good things in moderation. . . .

No matter how new or advanced you are in the workout department, you do not want to do too much too soon. Just as we don't want you to have an "all or nothing" mindset when it comes to dieting, the same applies to working out. You want to foster and nurture a lifelong love of exercise by doing activities that you adore so that working out never really feels like "work." With that said, though, your body and mind need balance when it comes to exercise, so you just can't keep doing the same one activity all the time for all time. You gotta mix things up! Keep these tips in mind for keeping your workouts balanced.

1. **IF IT'S SORE, GIVE IT A BREAK.** Your muscles need 24 to 48 hours to repair and rebuild after you've worked them. So if you wake up one morning and are super sore, it's best to choose a workout that doesn't directly work that body part. Of course, if that soreness happens every time you work out, then you need to take the intensity down a notch. Be sure that you're taking a few minutes to stretch before and after your workout; stretching when you wake up sore can do a world of good as well. But soreness—in moderation—isn't a bad thing; it's a sign that you're challenging yourself!

2. **SWITCH UP YOUR ROUTINE MONTHLY.** If variety is the spice of life, monotony is where all good workout intentions go to die. Do not fall

into the trap of doing the same thing over and over. Not only will it be boring after a few weeks, but you'll probably stop seeing results— and you're going to end up with an unbalanced bod!

3. **PLAN YOUR WORKOUTS AHEAD OF TIME.** It is much easier to have balance in your workouts if, in advance, you carve out time for what you want to do. Pick the times of day and days of the week that are going to be your nonnegotiable exercise times, and work the rest of your schedule around that. Write it down on your calendar. In ink.

4. **TAKE ONE TO TWO DAYS OFF A WEEK FROM FORMAL WORKOUTS.** Yes, you can get too much of a good thing! That's why we recommend taking a full day—or two—off formal workouts altogether each week (just not on back-to-back days if possible). In fact, working out too much has been linked to poor mood, impaired immunity, injury, and even stoppage in the results and performance department. While getting too much exercise probably isn't an issue for most of us, a day or two off a week is still essential. The break will keep you fresh and loving exercise—and works more moderation and balance into your life by giving you the flexibility to better flow with life without needing to get sweaty every darn day. It's all about making it doable and livable!

Now, we know that you're going to have to miss workouts now and again, and you won't always get that perfect mix of cardio, strength, and flexibility work in a week—and that's okay! When this happens, the key is not to throw in the towel and declare yourself worthless. Instead, it's a time to get creative and see how your bad-ass self can still squeeze in a little extra activity or stretching here or there. (P.S.: We didn't create those 10-minute workouts at the end of Chapter 3 for nothing—use 'em!)

ENERGIZE!
How Getting Out in Nature Is Good for the Soul

Need a burst of energy? Get yourself outside for a pick-me-up from Mother Nature herself. Studies have shown that getting active outdoors can have mental health benefits in addition to the physical ones, like lowering stress and anxiety, above and beyond what you'd get simply by working out at the gym. One study showed that even five minutes can have a significant impact on self-esteem and mood—and that if the green space also includes water like a river or lake, the effect is greater. So next time you're feeling unbalanced or stressed about an upcoming project, get yourself outside for a quick boost. If you usually work out indoors, try to take one of your weekly workouts to the great outdoors with a jog or bike ride, a hike in the woods, or even a game of Frisbee. Make getting yourself out of the house—and out of the gym—a priority for a natural high!

Balance All the Things

Just like with your foods and workouts, we want you to do the things you enjoy, that bring you energy, and that leave you with a zest for life! Start paying attention to what is and isn't working for you. Is saying yes to every request leaving you feeling burned out? Do you have people in your life who suck the energy right out of you? Are you getting enough time to yourself to just veg out and be alone? To focus on your own hobbies and interests? Start paying attention to the things that make you happy.

Does this mean you can shirk all of those things that zap you? Of course not. Things like taxes and work and certain obligations are necessary evils. But if certain things are bringing you down daily, look for ways to give yourself a break. If work is a major stressor, make it a point to step away for a lunch meditation break. If you have a hard time calling it a day and it has you burning the midnight oil, set a time when you call it quits and give yourself a break to relax and get your needed sleep. Does your weekly obligation with a friend wear you out? Maybe set up a monthly coffee date rather than a weekly dinner out. Does your Friday-night happy hour turn into many happy hours and leave you in recovery mode for half the weekend? Make adjustments as needed!

Only you know the things in your life that truly bring you energy and joy. So stand back and take inventory of your life, and try to get more of them while eliminating the energy-draining parts. Find what works best for you and do it!

Balance fixes

Feel like you're tipping over? It's time to get balanced! These 10-Minute Fixes will help you figure out what balance would look like in your daily life and give you steps to achieve that elusive beast. From carving out time for yourself to combating diet sabotage and learning to just say no, each fix is designed to make your life work for you!

1 **VISUALIZE A BALANCED YOU.** It's easy to hope, wish, and pray for more balance in your life when you're feeling out of whack. But try to turn that ideal of balance into concrete, tangible action items. It's basically like goal-setting: you want the end result—balance—but you need to know what to do to get there. That's where this fix comes in.

Remember how you created your Superhero Alter Ego back in Chapter 1? We want you to do the same thing here, only this time you're creating a healthy, balanced you. Take four minutes to do a mini meditation, and walk yourself through a day of being balanced. What does balance look like for you? How do you feel? What activities are you enjoying? What does an ideal balanced day look like for you? An ideal balanced week? What do your meals look like? What do your workouts look like? How is your energy?

After the four minutes is up, jot down any aha moments you had. Is there anything you can change in your life today to achieve more balance? What areas of your life aren't getting enough attention? What areas are getting too much attention? Review your notes of this balanced version of you so that you can check back in with your ideal balanced self when you feel yourself getting stressed. And even begin to make some small changes to your daily life to regain balance. Consider this exercise your touchstone so that when life gets crazy, you can remember what you're aiming for.

(2) **PLAN "ME TIME."** Carving out time for yourself isn't a luxury, it's a necessity. Your workouts and "me time" should feel like unbreakable appointments you have with yourself instead of things you do after all of your other responsibilities have been crossed off the list. Once you get into the habit of making yourself a priority, it'll just get easier! So once a week, take 10 minutes to gear up for the upcoming week. Get your calendar or grab your smartphone and plug in appointments with yourself. Pencil in that new cardio class you want to take. Schedule time to hit the salon for that relaxing pedicure you need. If you know you have a super-busy day of nonstop obligations, plan to start your day with a quick yoga session to clear your mind. Even taking five minutes to step away from your email and quietly enjoy a hot cup of tea or a slightly longer shower can do wonders for your mood.

If you find it's nearly impossible to get a moment alone, or any downtime at all, start carving more "me time" out of your everyday obligations. Make an energizing playlist or pick inspiring podcasts to listen to during your work commute. Add some of your favorite tunes to your least favorite tasks, like cleaning, cooking dinner, or grocery shopping. Take a break at work to look out the window for a boost from natural sunlight—do it for a full 60 seconds and you'll be amazed at how much more focused you are when you go back to your to-do list.

(3) **CREATE A BALANCED WORKOUT SCHEDULE.** A balanced workout schedule can do wonders for your life and your body, and creating one isn't nearly as hard as you might think. In fact, you're probably going to do it in less than 10 minutes. Booyah. So grab your calendar (digital or paper) and let's do it, step by step (Oh, baby—Gonna get to you, girl . . .).

Step 1: Block out the following chunks of time on your weekly calendar, based on what you've got going on and, if possible, placing them during times of the day when you have the most energy. Give yourself at least one or two days a week when you have no exercise scheduled. If you're a workout newbie or are pressed for time, go for the shorter amounts of time. If you're more seasoned or have the wiggle room in your schedule, go for longer! And feel free to layer these or separate them throughout the day, making sure that no one day has more than 70 minutes total. Choose the combination that works best for you!

- Three 30- to 60-minute segments of time
- Two 10- to 30-minute segments of time
- Five 5- to 10-minute blocks a week

Step 2: Now, go through and place the following workouts for your blocks. Try to equally place them so that you're not doing the same type of workout on back-to-back days, except for stretching. (See? Told you this would be easy.)

- **Three 30- to 60-minute segments of time:** Two cardio workouts and one strength workout
- **Two 10- to 30-minute segments of time:** One high-intensity interval workout and one circuit-training strength workout

- **Five 5- to 10-minute blocks a week:** Stretch or yoga (whichever you feel like and enjoy more!)

Step 3: Next, pick out exactly what workouts you'll be doing. And pick out workouts that get you excited to do them. If you're blanking on ideas, head on back to Chapter 3 for 10-minute workouts to incorporate!

(4) **PRACTICE SAYING NO.** We've been working on the wonderful things you can add to your life to help you achieve balance—delicious foods, awesome workouts. But sometimes there are things you need to nix. Sometimes you just have to say no.

If you're a people-pleaser by nature, it can be a real challenge to say no to someone. It's easier to just go along with it rather than ruffle any feathers. But learning to say no can go a long way to achieving balance in your life. Plus, it'll help when you are dealing with any of the saboteurs we'll talk about later. Think back to the last few times you've said yes to a commitment when you wanted to say no. Put yourself back in that situation and practice saying no. Whether it's someone asking you about a social obligation you don't want to make, someone tempting you to skip a workout, or someone bringing you another beer you didn't want, stick to your guns.

So practice actually saying it out loud. No. No! Walk yourself through a few scenarios when it may be really hard to say no. Picture yourself actually doing it and saying it—and feeling empowered for doing so. It may feel weird and unfamiliar at first, but just like any muscle, it gets stronger the more you practice. Then make it a goal to say no the next time you need to.

10-Minute Fixes

Here are a few scenarios to practice:

- "Want to come out for a few drinks?" "No, thanks, I'm busy tonight."
- "You should come to my son's first birthday party! It's all day long on Saturday!" "Thanks for the invite, but, no, I'm not able to make it!"
- "Want to go out to dinner with me?" "No, thank you."
- "One missed workout won't hurt; come out for dessert instead!" "No."

You don't have to make excuses, and you don't have to make up lies. It will get easier, we promise.

(5) **QUENCH A CRAVING THE HEALTHY WAY.** We're all human, therefore we all get cravings. And denying them is a surefire way to end up feeling deprived. Plus, ignoring a craving can turn it into an obsession and give a food power it doesn't deserve—not exactly an ideal and balanced situation. Being an FBG means allowing yourself to have the foods you love in reasonable quan- tities, allowing you to keep ice cream in the house without being afraid you'll eat the entire gallon!

For some people, cravings come in the form of that sweet tooth that perks up every night at 9 P.M. For others, it's a salt craving each afternoon. For others it's more about texture—the crunch of a chip or the smooth creaminess of pudding. Maybe you don't discriminate when it comes to your cravings and they change on a daily basis. But cravings can take up a dispropor- tionate amount of mental energy if you feel that you have to constantly do battle with them; trying to ignore a craving for some potato chips or ice cream is going to leave you thinking about those foods a lot more than if you'd had a taste when the craving first struck you. If you can look forward to a glass of wine and a piece of dark chocolate at the end of the day, you probably won't spend the whole day thinking about how bummed you are that you don't get to have those things!

We are not about to tell you that anything is off-limits when it comes to your cravings, but we do want you to look at precisely what you're craving before you head off to quench it. We want you to commit to the craving so you can satisfy it appropriately, instead of grazing on everything in the kitchen and feeling like you're still missing that "little something." Next time that craving hits, take 10 minutes to really examine it. Decode your craving by asking yourself the following questions:

- Why do I need it right now? Is there a healthier alternative that could fulfill the same need, or a way that I can integrate some extra nutrition into my craving?
- What am I craving specifically? Do I want a taste, like sweet, salty, sour, or savory? Or a texture, like crunchy, smooth, creamy? A temperature—warm, hot, cold, or frozen? Is it a specific food item?
- How much will it take to truly satisfy my desire?

Say, for instance, you're craving a piece of thick white toast smothered with peanut butter and honey. First, are you actually bored? Missing your mom, who always made that snack for you when you were young? Or are you truly hungry? If you decide you're hungry, carry on. Can you be satisfied with a healthier whole-grain bread? Wheat bread? A few whole-grain crackers?

If so, will a thin spread of peanut butter and a little drizzle of honey satisfy you instead of huge globs of both? Make your snack, put it on a plate, and put everything away before you take your first bite. Then really enjoy and savor it!

It's important to decide on your craving before you even head into the kitchen, particularly if you've been a chronic mindless muncher in the past. Plus, mentally preparing for your craving will make it all the more satisfying!

No matter how you set about satisfying those cravings—the full-fat real deal or a modified lightened-up version you've found—be mindful of portions. Ever notice how the first few bites of anything are the most delicious? We thought so. Enjoying a small serving of ice cream will probably give you the same thrill as downing an entire pint of ice cream, without the nasty side effect of a stomachache. And remember that just because something is "light" doesn't mean you can eat twice as much. Sharing is caring—and consider that you're sharing today's treat with your tomorrow self.

(6) **RESEARCH THE HEALTHIEST OPTIONS AT YOUR FAVORITE RESTAURANTS.** It's so easy to be a creature of habit when it comes to dining out. You found that dish you love at your favorite restaurant and you order it every time. We're not saying you can never have it again. But if you know it's not the healthiest option (Waves hi to fish and chips! High-fives fettuccine Alfredo!), this fix is about seeking out other healthier and more balanced options to try.

In the next 10 minutes, make a list of your five favorite restaurants—the ones you hit up the most frequently. Then take thee to the Internet and pull up the menu for each one. See if they have a light menu. Investigate menu items that sound yummy and are on the lighter side. Write down (or make a note on your smartphone) the several healthier options for each restaurant. Then, no matter how tempting your favorite meal sounds when you sit down to dine, order something on your pre-approved list. This can be a fantastic way to discover new favorites, and we promise you'll be pleasantly surprised at how tasty healthy options can be!

Once you've checked all of your regular joints, seek out five new restaurants to try and do the same menu research for each one. Challenge yourself to get out of your comfort zone. Try new cuisine you haven't experienced; ethnic restaurants often have awesome healthy veggie-based dishes. The more you experiment, the longer your list of healthy dining options will be. Variety truly is the spice of life—and healthy eating!

(7) **LEARN YOUR PORTION BASICS.** Sure, you've read the nutrition label. You know a proper portion of ice cream is half a cup. You know a serving of peanut butter is two tablespoons. But do you know what those actually *look* like? In this quick fix, you're going to take 10 minutes to get familiar with all of those measurements again and get your portion sizes balanced!

Head to your kitchen and pull out your measuring cups and spoons, as well as a bowl and plate you usually use. Then you'll need a few different edibles to measure, like uncooked rice, pasta, cereal or oatmeal, nuts or trail mix, and some fruit, like grapes or chopped apple or pear. Also grab a couple of common cooking ingredients, like oil and sugar or flour.

10-Minute Fixes

Now start playing with your food. Measure out a cup of cereal and dish it into your bowl. Put half a cup of pasta on your plate. See what a cup of berries looks like. Compare a serving of grapes to a serving of raisins; which would be a more filling snack? Check out a serving of trail mix or nuts. Measure out two tablespoons of oil and see what that looks like so you can get an idea of how much to throw in a skillet. Hold a tablespoon of sugar in the palm of your hand so you can see how much that is. The idea here is to get a visual of what different measurements mean: What does a cup or a tablespoon actually look like on your plate or in your bowl?

We certainly don't want you to start measuring everything that goes into your mouth, and you don't need to pull out your measuring cup every time you munch on some tortilla chips. But having a mental snapshot of the proper serving size will better keep your eats in balance and help you eyeball it more accurately when you're cooking or grabbing a snack. Taking this 10 minutes now will actually save you time in the long run.

(8) SEE IF YOU'RE REALLY LIVING THE 80/20 PRINCIPLE. The 80/20 principle is fantastic in theory, but it sometimes can be a bit deceiving to follow, as 20 percent of the food you eat is hard to visualize. So that's what this 10-Minute Fix helps with! Follow these steps to make sure your 20 percent isn't actually 30 percent or 40 percent—or that you're not giving yourself enough wiggle room!

Instead of looking at each meal as 80/20, which can get tricky to track, look at a full week of eats. That way, if you want to go out for margaritas and chips and salsa with your girlfriends on Friday night, you totally can and make that part of your 20 percent weekly balance. Yes, we know there's math involved, but you can do it!

Step 1: Figure out how many meals you eat a week. This will be 21 for most of us, although if you do the mini-meal thing (which can be awesome if it works for you!), it may be more. Now, if you're a snacker and would rather use your 20 percent just for snacks, then count how many snacks you have in a typical week.

Step 2: Find your 20 percent. Once you have your number from step 1, multiply it by 0.2. For 21 meals, that's 4.2. This means that you can incorporate your favorite less-than-healthy foods in your meals about four times a week. If you used snacks instead of meals, take your number from step 1 and take it times 0.2. That is, if you normally have 14 snacks in a week, you'll get 2.8 (14 x 0.2). Double that for a total of 5.6 snackaroos to play with.

And if you'd like to use your 20 percent on both meals *and* snacks? Well, take your meals number and cut it in half to figure out your 20 percent for meals (in the previous example, 2.1), and then double that halved number for your percentage of snacks (4.2).

Now, that's assuming that you are also following your hunger, really savoring and enjoying each delicious bite, and still trying to eat meals with a nice balance of protein, fiber, and healthy fat. But that's quite a bit of wiggle room to play with, right? And totally doable!

"If you change the way you look at things, the things you look at change."

—DR. WAYNE DYER

9 DO A BALANCE WORKOUT. We've been talking this whole chapter about the concept of balance, but ya'll know the physical aspect of balance, too, right? The one where you're able to stand on one foot with your eyes closed and hop up and down without falling over? Or walking on a tightrope? Or master that complicated yoga pose where you get your feet above your head? Yep, that balance. Thankfully, in order to have better balance, you don't have to do any of that crazy stuff. (Although you can, for fun, if you want.) Instead, you can just do this 10-minute balancing workout!

Warm-up: Take three deep breaths to center and focus yourself.

Standing leg raises: From a standing position, lift your right knee up and hold for 30 seconds. Then extend your leg out straight in front of you for another 30 seconds. Lower your leg back down to the ground. Repeat sequence on your left leg.

Standing leg raises challenge: If that was challenging, do the standing leg raises on each side again. If it wasn't, grab a pillow and place it below your standing foot. Try the standing leg raises again. (Harder, huh?)

Airplane: Get down on the floor in an all-fours position. Extend your right arm up and out in front of you. Once you have your balance, extend your left leg out and back behind you. Hold for as long as you can, working up to one minute. Repeat on the other side.

Airplane challenge: If you couldn't finish a full minute in airplane, do another set of the basic version. If you can, make it harder by reaching your hands and feet not just out in front of and behind you, but have them reach out to the side for extra balance work. Ah, yeah!

Cool-down: Take three more deep breaths, repeating the phrase *I am balanced and healthy*. Feel good!

(10) **JOURNAL YOUR RESPONSE:** *What balance means to me.* We keep saying that *balance* means different things to different people. But what it means to *you* is the most important definition of all. That's why for this journal assignment, you are to explore what the word means to you—in *all* areas of your life. Set a timer for 10 minutes, grab that journal, and let the thoughts flow. Think about how balance applies to your day-to-day life. How important is balance to you? What roles do your career, family, friendships, hobbies, workouts, and nutrition play? How can you naturally feel more balanced? The question may seem simple, but we guarantee you'll probably learn something new about how this concept applies to you—and how you can begin to feel more balanced!

CHAPTER 5

Focus on the Positives

....

Being an FBG isn't just about eating this or doing that workout: it's truly a state of mind about all areas of your life. It's the thoughts we think, the lens we choose to see through, and the energy and attitude we bring to every facet of our lives. No matter what you weigh or what size clothes you wear, you won't be able to enjoy your physical life if you're not also living an emotionally satisfying one. A life that you choose to love and embrace. Because it doesn't matter how many workouts you do or how many healthy foods you eat; if you're truly not enjoying your life and seeing all the good in the world, then you're not going to be able to sustain all of the habits that make up the FBG lifestyle for a lifetime!

We know that being positive is sometimes easier said than done. It's easy to feel bogged down and focus on all of the things that *aren't* going right in your life. From money, to work, to busy schedules, to all of the terrible stuff you see on the 5 o'clock news, there is a lot to fret over. But we'll give you the tools to lift some of that mental weight off of your shoulders so that you can begin to see and embrace the positive in your life and the world.

The old question "Do you see the glass half full or half empty?" may be an overused measure of attitude, but it's an awfully good one. And in this chapter, we help you flip your thinking to see and focus on all the good you've got going on in your life. We help you to identify the areas of your life that might be the hardest for you when trying a new approach to healthy living—and once you've figured out what those tricky areas are, you'll be ready to figure out ways to alleviate them!

Retrain Your Brain

If all of this positive-attitude talk has you rolling your eyes and saying, "Come on, FBGs, this is *sooo* cheesy," take note: although we generally find that people seem to be happier when they focus on the good in their lives, it's also been studied quite a bit. And what scientists have found has been pretty amazing. Not only does thinking positive thoughts and focusing on the good boost self-confidence, but it can also help with weight loss and workouts. One study found that women who wrote about the things they valued most in life each day lost more weight than those who didn't, and another study found that people who lifted weights with positive action verbs—like I *lift* the dumbbell instead of I *don't lift* the dumbbell—had better grip strength than those who heard negative talk.

Both of these studies point to the power of the word. People say that "sticks and stones may break my bones, but words will never hurt me," but that's just not true. The words we use and the thoughts we have *do* have power. Incredible power. The thoughts we think over and over actually begin to develop into emotions that we feel. As we begin to feel a certain way, then we start to act out from that emotion. And as we begin to act out of an emotion over time, we can develop habits with our behaviors. So a behavior or unhealthy habit that seems to come out of nowhere is actually rooted in thought. Here are a few examples:

Repeated thought: *I hate my job.*
Resulting emotion: Anger, frustration, anxiety
Resulting behavior: Impatience, impulsive decisions
Resulting unhealthy habit: Ordering unhealthy foods when out, drinking too much to relax

Repeated thought: *I'm not good enough.*
Resulting emotion: Sadness, loneliness
Resulting behavior: Reluctant to do new things, lack of energy to work out
Resulting unhealthy habit: Won't eat certain healthy foods, aversion to exercise

Repeated thought: *Life isn't fair.*
Resulting emotion: Powerlessness, fear
Resulting behavior: Playing the victim, being a martyr
Resulting unhealthy habit: Giving up too easily during workouts, making excuses to not take care of yourself because you have to care for others

When you get right down to it, all we really are is our thoughts. Our perceptions of and our thoughts about the world determine how we react to it and what behaviors we respond with. Over time, those behaviors that we repeat become habits. Habits that, as we discussed, can be tough to break. Left in place long enough, habits become values and key beliefs that we have about ourselves. Our thoughts basically become a self-fulfilling prophecy—whether we think we can or cannot do something, we're right.

So if that's how powerful our own thoughts can be, what about when those ideas are reinforced by the culture around us? While there is always a new diet, a new workout, and a new magical solution to weight problems around the corner, the overwhelming message that we get when we start talking about weight loss is that it's going to be *hard*. And so we psych ourselves out about it before we've even begun. Making the time to prepare a healthy meal is hard because we *think* it is. But couldn't we really turn off the TV 10 minutes earlier and chop some veggies for the next day (or plop a cutting board down in front of the TV)? Sure. Could we start ordering healthier meals when we go out and be excited about all the good things that food is going to do for us? Abso-freakin'-lutely.

And this is where the power of positive thinking really comes into play. No matter what your goals are, you have to start to become aware of your thoughts. Are they setting you up for success or are they leading you down a path of negative emotions, behaviors, and unhealthy habits? Over the course of a day, start to pay attention to what's going on in your head. Then see how you can flip it for the positive. Could you focus on what you *do* like about your job instead of what you dislike about it? Could you remind yourself that you are worthy of taking care of? Could you learn to better appreciate the natural ebb and flow that is life? Again, some examples!

Repeated thought: *I am thankful for my job.*
Resulting emotion: Satisfaction, gratefulness

Resulting behavior: Calm, patient
Resulting healthy habit: Thinks before ordering, more mindful when eating and drinking

Repeated thought: *I can do anything I set my mind to.*
Resulting emotion: Empowered, confident
Resulting behavior: Willing to try new things, energetic
Resulting healthy habit: Experiments with new healthy foods and recipes, challenges herself with new workouts

Repeated thought: *Life is a beautiful journey.*
Resulting emotion: Curiosity, excitement
Resulting behavior: Willingness to learn, being adventurous
Resulting healthy habit: Not giving up or expecting perfection from herself, being a leader and inspiring others

Perception is everything. How you view your life and what you tell yourself in your head is and will continue to be your reality. Yes, we know crappy things happen and that you can't always be 100 percent happy all the time. And that's fine—we don't want you to be a perfect perky Pollyanna; we want you to be real. But we definitely want you to focus on the good as much as you can and challenge yourself to start seeing the positives of not only your healthy lifestyle but also your entire life.

Remember, living a healthy lifestyle isn't about what you "have to" or "can't" do. It's about the "get-tos"! This is not a diet; it's about giving yourself permission to go and find the things you love. It's about looking objectively at all areas of your life, examining your thoughts and beliefs and digging deep and being brave to break through your own barriers to try new things that you might love.

It's about letting go of all of those negative thoughts and beliefs you have. It's about making changes at the root cause (aka your thoughts) of your issues and replacing them with positive ones. This is how you drop the mental and emotional weight that has been holding you back from making healthy permanent changes in your life. This is what it means to be an FBG!

Get Grateful

We all have sooo much to be grateful for. The fact that you even had the money to buy this book or the access to a library to check it out is something to be thankful for. Let alone that you have the education to know how to read it! And we'd be willing to put money on the fact that you're probably sitting there with a cell phone next to you, and with running water and electricity. That makes you already luckier than millions of people around the world! Think of that the next time you're seriously bummed that your favorite sports team lost, or you—gasp!—gained a pound. Talk about reframing your thoughts, huh?

But having an attitude of gratitude isn't just about focusing on how much worse it could be; it's also about just looking around and being amazed by what you see and even what your body can do. It's about feeling the sunshine on your cheeks when you're outside. It's in the smile on your loved one's face. It's within a really good meal you're about to eat. Heck, it's even about a warm cup of coffee in the morning and having a comfy blanket to snuggle up in at night. It's about the big things, the little things, and the everyday things. Just look around you and begin to notice all of the things you are thankful for. The list is endless! (And to get your gratitude attitude going, check out our 10-Minute Fixes at the end of the chapter!)

An attitude of gratitude has huge health gains, too. Practicing thankfulness has been linked to feeling less anxious and depressed; it can leave you feeling healthier, well rested, and with higher long-term satisfaction with life. In fact, researchers from the University of California, Davis, found that just keeping a journal listing five things that you're grateful for—like a pretty sunset or a kind gesture from a friend—with just a sentence about each, left people feeling more optimistic and happier after just two weeks. Those who kept a gratitude journal also spent more time working out.

The real secret to gratitude's power lies in how it makes you *feel*. When you sit down to think about what you're grateful for, you focus on the good, which makes you feel good. And when you feel good, you have more energy. You're less likely to self-medicate your emotions with unhealthy foods or pump yourself up with caffeine or sugar. You feel more fulfilled with your everyday life and are less likely to turn to food or TV to de-stress. Really, when you feel good, you tend to make healthier, better-for-you decisions! So don't just get thankful on Thanksgiving, get an attitude of gratitude 365 days a year!

Working Out: Positively Beautiful

If sweating up a storm and pumping iron don't fit your typical idea of beauty and positivity, we want to turn your preconceived notions on their head! Sure, not all workouts are positively beautiful and inspiring. Sometimes you'll be frustrated or sore, and the workout will just be hard—and you'll feel far from beautiful. Or you're clumsy or you trip. And that's okay! Don't let your uncooperative body or a bad day at the gym get in your head.

We always say to talk to yourself as if you're talking to your best friend. You'd never give a friend a hard time for having to take a break to catch her breath. You'd never snark on your bud's bod while she's doing deadlifts. You'd never think your pal was a failure because she couldn't do a regular push-up. So don't do those things to yourself!

Train your brain to focus on the positive during your workouts: You're working out! You're getting fit! You're dripping with delicious sweat. (Eww.) You're doing amazing things with your body. You might think you look silly doing it, but who's watching? And more important, who cares? Our bodies were made to move, even if you're tripping your way through a dance DVD or trying not to fall off an exercise bike. Give yourself pep talks as you work out. Any time you feel a negative comment pop into your brain, replace it with a positive one. If you're out of breath, focus on how great it's going to feel when you get to the next break. If you're frustrated that you're not picking up the moves, slow down until you feel you've gotten it right. There is no wrong way to get physical, and beating yourself up is never allowed in the FBG world. If you need help being positive during workouts, try our affirmation workout in our quick fixes!

Want one solution to help you feel more beautiful in your workouts? Do beautiful workouts! To balance your heart-pumping, sweat-inducing workout sessions that don't feel especially gorgeous, try dance, Pilates, and barre classes that will have you embracing your inner dancer—the fluid, graceful goddess you have inside! As with everything else in life, you can only improve your coordination, agility, and grace if you work at them. These types of workouts might not make you a super ballerina, but they will improve your posture, body awareness, and core strength—all of which go a long way toward helping you incorporate gracefulness into your everyday life. Or, at least, less clumsiness!

"A positive attitude causes a chain reaction of positive thoughts, events, and outcomes. It is a catalyst and it sparks extraordinary results."

—WADE BOGGS

Love Your Food

So many of us say that we "love food." But take a second and think about if you *really* treat your food with love. Do some foods scare you because you feel as if you have no self-control around them? Do you really enjoy your food—or do you scarf it down while rushing from one to-do to the next? Or are you nibbling over the sink? (Yes, we know eating over the sink saves you from washing a dish, but it's not worth it. Promise.) Worse yet, are you secretly eating and feeling ashamed of your actions? All of these examples—and we've all done them before!—aren't really acts of food-love and respect.

Really pay attention to the way you eat and the thoughts you bring to the experience. Challenge yourself to always sit down with a plate and honor your time eating. Be grateful for what's on your plate and think positively about how good that food is going to make you feel.

Remind yourself that you are worth taking care of and continue

ORGANIC, VEGAN, FREE-RANGE . . . SAY WHA?

There are about a million different labels on foods these days. From non-GMO, to vegan-friendly, to gluten-free, to organic, to free-range, to cage-free, and everything in between; it's enough to make a gal's healthy head spin. From conflicting news stories to your co-worker telling you that organic is the *only* way to go, we have just one piece of advice: do what works for you and eat in a way that feels right and makes sense. You already have our guidelines for eating healthy (eat when you're hungry, stop when you're full, and eat all good things in moderation and with balance). But beyond that, you are the one who gets to decide what you enjoy eating and what feels best for your body and your morals. If that's vegan, awesome. If it's gluten-free, go for it. If it's organic 100 percent of the time, knock yourself out. Heck, you may not even need a label like "vegetarian" or "Paleo" at all! You may just find that you're in a category all your own.

focusing on the positives that your healthy life is bringing you. While food is awesome, remember that most of those times when we're eating out or are at social occasions, the purpose of the gathering goes deeper than just what's on the menu. It's about connecting with others, spending time with those you love, and enjoying the conversation and experience. So don't get caught up on what you "can't" eat. Remember to focus on what you "get to" eat, and then spend your time enjoying yourself for the real reason you're there.

What You See Is What You Get

Now that you're starting to see the importance of eating, working out, and seeing the world in a more positive light, we want to take you to the next level: the environment. Yes, you can—as we've recommended—begin to see your current situation and choices in a more uplifting, feel-good way, but also begin to seek out the goodness.

In addition to eating healthy foods and doing workouts that bring you energy, think of what other forces are at play in your life. How often do your friends lift you up or bring you down? Are you listening to music that makes you feel happy and joyful, or are your tunes kind of angry or depressing? How do the movies and TV shows you watch make you feel? Do you love the colors in your home?

It can be easy to go through the motions of your day without being fully aware of the experience. Just think of how many times you've driven somewhere only to realize that you were off in your own world and not really paying attention to driving. (Yeah, it freaks us out when it happens, too.) But take an objective look at *all* areas of your life, from your daily routines, to your relationships, to your media usage, to your décor. We all have little routines and rituals we follow every day. Here are a few tweaks to make yours a little happier.

Morning: Do you begin your day with a loud, annoying alarm? Well, that obviously sets a negative tone for the morning. Try swapping it out for a more calming, natural sound to wake up to, like chirping birds. Or try one of those alarms that use light to trigger you out of sleep. Oh, and are you rushing around in the morning? Not the best headspace to start the day. Give yourself plenty of time in the morning to get ready and out the door so that you're not rushed from the get-go.

Afternoon: Our natural energy rhythms tend to dip in the afternoon. This is why it's important to eat a balanced and nutritious lunch, stay hydrated, and have a healthy snack on hand for the afternoon hours. And instead of beating yourself up for wanting to take a nap at 3 P.M., cut yourself some slack and plan a little downtime, like doing an easy task at work or even taking a five-minute chat break with a friend or co-worker. Part of being an FBG is working with what your mama (or evolution) gave ya, not working against it.

Evening: Many of us fall into the habit of mindlessly munching in front of the telly after dinner, which can thwart our healthy living goals and make us feel that we're not in control of our eating habits. So instead of reaching for chips, snuggle up with a cup of caffeine-free tea. And make a point of having at least an hour between your bedtime and your screen time. This switch alone will make you sleep better and feel better about yourself and your choices.

FROM THE FBGs
How to Bust Out of a Bad Mood

FROM ERIN: Oh, the bad moods. They hit everyone, and I'm certainly not immune. But when the grumpies strike, I strike back. And usually, I win. Or at least give them a black eye. Here's how.

1. *I get outside.* Nothing cures a bad mood like going outdoors. Whether it's simply to take a walk around the block, sit on the back porch, or kick a ball around the backyard with my kids, getting into the sun is a major mood booster. I even weirdly enjoy yardwork because it gets me outside. The sunbeam effect has also been studied; there are scientific reasons you're happier out in the sun!

2. *I vent away.* I try to bust a bad mood with a little complaining. For me, talking out my frustrations and funkiness is a surefire

way to get some relief from my grumpitude. Whether I email, text, or call my husband, a friend, or family member to complain, I certainly feel better when I get it off my chest. But I don't just complain about the same frustrations over and over; I use venting as a pressure release, a way to blow off steam before moving on and doing what I can to change what's frustrating me.

3. *I have a phone pick-me-up.* A sure way to distract myself from a foul mood is to grab my phone and browse through my pictures and videos. Photos and funny videos of family, pets, and friends always bring back fun memories and put a smile on my face.

4. *I nap.* I know myself well enough by now to have figured out that my grumpiness is often the direct result of a lack of sleep. If I can swing it, even a 10-minute nap or quiet time while the kids are napping goes a long way to picking my mood off the ground.

5. *I "Britney."* Okay, so it doesn't always have to be Britney Spears, but I definitely have those songs that just put me in a good mood. It's hard not to be in a good mood when certain songs come on. So I pump up the jam. The pop-music jam!

Not feeling positive yet? Want to feel more positive? Want us to convince you that the glass really is half full—maybe even almost completely full? These 10-Minute Fixes will have you focused on the positive and awesome in your life. You'll have positivity coming out of your ears. In a good way!

1. **LIST ALL THE HEALTHY THINGS YOU LOVE.** Take 10 minutes to write down all the healthy things you've ever loved, from workouts, to active pastimes, to foods. This list should include fruits and veggies that you like, regardless of the last time you had them. Be sure to write down anything active you enjoy that doesn't involve sitting on the couch. List any new healthy-living discoveries that you've tried or have been curious about. Use this as an opportunity to focus on all of the awesomeness you've added to your life already, and to serve as a reminder of new things that are ahead of you. After all, it's awesome that you've discovered kale and not totally heartbreaking that you've decided it's best to bypass french fries most of the time. And it's awesome that you've taken up biking—we doubt your couch misses you for that hour you aren't there!

   Use this list of healthy awesomeness as inspiration the next time you're feeling unmotivated. Bring it to the grocery store the next time you feel you're in a food rut; use it at the gym or when you're feeling bored to keep those favorite workouts and activities top-of-mind. As you find new healthy stuff you love, add it to your list. We suggest trying Zumba and roasted Brussels sprouts.

2. **PLAN TO DO SOMETHING YOU LOVE.** Busy, busy, busy. We're all so busy that it can feel as if there is just no time for fun. But

we want you to plan that downtime! Just as you plan your workout schedule, we want you to schedule (in pencil, or marker, or digital form) an appointment to do something you love or to do something you've always wanted to try. It doesn't have to be fitness-related, but it does have to be something that brings you joy. Maybe you've played piano for years and gotten away from it lately. Set aside an hour to tickle the ivories! Maybe you've been an avid knitter but haven't touched a ball of yarn in years. Make a date with yourself to hit a craft store and get supplies for your next project. That friend who makes you laugh uncontrollably? Make a date with her. Your favorite movie that makes you giggle? Set aside an afternoon this weekend to watch it. Or go to the movie theater to see that guilty-pleasure film you've had your eye on; solo movie excursions can be a lot of fun.

As we said in the last chapter, balance in all areas in your life is key, so don't get away from your other loves just because you're putting a lot of time and energy into increasing your cardio and pushing your push-ups to the next level. Being an FBG means loving your life, not just working hard for a hot bod!

(3) **CREATE A FEEL-GOOD MORNING RITUAL.** Some people jump out of bed in the morning, ready to take on the day—even if it means getting out of bed before 6 A.M. for workouts (ahem, Jenn). Others are not morning people and hit the snooze button about a million times before dragging themselves out of bed and/ or avoid social interactions for at least 30 minutes while they wake up (ahem, Erin). If the latter sounds more like you, we've got a morning feel-good ritual that will help ease you into the A.M.

First, when you wake up, avoid hitting the snooze button. You have 10 minutes to do this fix, and the snooze would blow it. While you're still lying down, stretch your body lengthwise as long and as tall as you can. Put your arms above your head, and stretch all the way down to your feet. Take a full minute for this stretch; wiggle your fingers and your toes. Flex and point your feet. Breathe deeply the whole time.

Now sit up with your legs comfortably crossed. Stretch your arms high above your head, and with your hands clasped, lean side to side as you breathe in and out. You should feel an awesome stretch through your sides. Still sitting, lift your arms up to your sides with your palms facing forward. Move your arms back as you slightly arch your back and bring your shoulder blades together. Reverse this move as you round your back forward.

Then, with the soles of your feet together and your knees out, lean over your feet to stretch your inner thighs for a moment. Next, put your feet straight in front of you for a hamstring stretch.

While you're stretching yourself awake, focus on getting into a positive mindset and set a healthy intention for the day. You should be energized enough to open the shades to let in natural light or flip on that light switch and face the day. You may never learn to love mornings, but at least this will make them just a tad more enjoyable. Plus, you can feel good that you've already done something to start your day off right before you even got out of bed—flexibility work! Now go get yourself a cup of coffee or tea; you're awake enough to really enjoy it!

(4) **MAKE A DREAM BOARD.** In FBG land, we're big on dreaming and goal-setting to be our best. Without goals, it's easy to just float along with no sense of purpose—in workouts and in life.

That's why we want you to create a dream board with images and words that inspire you and make you happy. It may seem silly, but you'll be amazed at the way looking at a dream board can bring a burst of inspiration to remind you of your hopes, dreams, and aspirations. It's a daily reminder to check in with the big picture, to remember that life isn't just about those mundane details that can drag you down!

So grab a piece of poster board or a bulletin board, a pair of scissors, and a few of your favorite magazines. Flip through the pages and cut out images that inspire: vacation destinations, meals that look delicious, activities you'd like to try, clothes you'd like to try on, words that you can use as motivational mantras. If it gives you a sense of pleasure, happiness, or satisfaction when you see it, get to clipping! Avoid anything that gives you anxiety or that brings up negativity—this board is purely positive.

Stick all of the images to the poster board or bulletin board and hang it somewhere you'll see it every day, such as in your office, or put it somewhere you can refer to it each morning, such as in your nightstand drawer. Fill the whole page up if you like, or leave space so you can add to it—you make the dream board rules. Maybe you'll decide to make a new one each year on your birthday or as the new year starts. Or, if you're feeling down in the dumps (winter can do that to the best of us), use that as a time to make a new one to inspire and get you through until spring!

(5) **DO YOUR WORKOUTS WITH AFFIRMATIONS.** Of the many interesting and notable workout DVDs we've tried and reviewed, one of the most memorable paired spoken affirmations with the workout. We thought that it might feel a little silly to be repeating positive phrases while following along with the exercises, but it actually made us smile and gave us an energy boost as we sweat. So we decided to create our own FBG-afied version! You can repeat these affirmations out loud or simply chant in a rhythm in your head. You be the judge of how accepting those around you are!

Pair these affirmations with the accompanying move as you do them during your regular workouts, or do each of these moves for one minute and repeat the circuit twice for an affirming quick 10-minute workout.

Boxer shuffle with jabs: *I am super strong; I will knock this out!*
Positive push-ups: *I am a push-up machine.*
Squats with jump: *I am a Fit Bottomed Girl!* (jump)
Biceps curls: *Just look at these guns; I work out.*
Jumping jacks: *Don't jack with me; I'm as strong as can be!*

You may have mantras pop into your head as you work out, so go with what's working for you, what makes you giggle, and what gets you to push yourself.

(6) **GIVE YOURSELF A MIDDAY PEP TALK.** Did you ever see the viral video of the little girl in the bathroom giving herself a pep talk before school? She lists all the things she loves, while dancing around on the countertop. Don't worry, we're not going to make you stand up on the countertop in your PJs, although we do want you to give yourself a pep talk with as much enthusiasm as that girl had. Whether you're standing in front of the mirror or in your car shouting your pep talk out loud, or if you're in the elevator at work or standing in line for lunch saying it in your head, any time is a good time for this pep talk. Don't even worry about taking a full 10 minutes; even just a few minutes of positivity directed at yourself will boost your mood.

Reserve this pep talk for days when you just aren't feeling like working out. Be your own cheerleader here and break out all of the spirit fingers you can imagine in your head. Or if the friendly cheerleader vibe doesn't work for you, break out your inner drill sergeant! Tell yourself how awesome you'll feel once you get that workout in. Tell yourself how this workout will help you achieve your goals and will give you the energy you need to face the rest of the day. Tell yourself you're going to break through mental barriers and set personal records. Plan the workout you want to do, and get mentally pumped for it!

Use this pep talk to get yourself in the right frame of mind. If you actively tell yourself that you *get* to work out—rather than *have to* work out, or *should* work out—you're going to be amazed at how your attitude about working out will actually change. It's a case of mind over matter!

7 **SET UP A GRATITUDE EMAIL OR TEXT EXCHANGE.** By now we hope we have you convinced of all the awesomeness that life has to offer and all the amazing things you should be grateful for. Positivity can be contagious, so arrange to share that positivity with a friend daily. Pick a friend—it can be your workout buddy

or a family member who is eternally optimistic—and set up a daily email gratitude exchange.

Each morning, share a line or two with your partner about what you're grateful for that day. Try to go at least a month (or a year!) before repeating anything, so as to force yourself to think outside the gratitude box and to recognize things both big and small. From a daily cup of warm tea, to having air-conditioning, to your dog being cute, there are literally a million things to say thank-you for!

Doing this exchange will force you to find positivity on even the bleakest, dreariest mornings. Plus, seeing the other person's text or email might remind you of another thing you can be grateful for in your day that you may not have noticed without that reminder. That daily connection can also bring a smile to your face, even on the roughest days, when you're bogged down in work and mundane obligations. That one moment guarantees that you connect with a friend and can set a positive tone for the rest of your day. So connect up, and get those feel-good vibes flowing!

(8) **CREATE A POSITIVE DINING EXPERIENCE.** So often meals are about necessity—I'm hungry, must fill up!—and we forget that they can be a beautiful *experience*. That's why this fix is all about creating a positive dining experience. For your next meal—whether it's a taco salad or the fanciest meal you have in your cooking repertoire—take 10 minutes to make it all about the beauty.

Get out your finest tablecloth. Grab the fine china (or the nicest dishes you have that don't have cracks! We know how that

10-Minute Fixes

goes.) and those special napkins you save for company. Dig out the crystal serving dishes. Dim the lights and light the candles. Put on soothing music for ambience.

Remember that *G* for gorgeous meals? Make it so! Pull out your inner diva chef and think about the presentation of your meal rather than just throwing it on a plate willy-nilly. When you take the time to cook and make the meal fabulous, you'll have a greater appreciation for the food. You'll take the time to savor it, from the look to the taste to the entire experience, and enjoy all of the fancy—even if it's on a Wednesday night.

(9) END THE DAY WITH A BRIGHT SPOT. Even the toughest days have a bright side. Though it may be hard to find sometimes, make a point to write down in a gratitude journal or log on your phone one bright spot each day as you're winding down before you hit the hay. It can be anything, but for a few minutes before you go to sleep, create a ritual of taking time to jot down a few sentences about something that made you smile that day.

Whether it was your perfect morning coffee that was rich and steamy or a compliment you got from your boss on a job well done, nothing is too big or too small to include. Look back on your day and find the brightest spot in it. Whether it's something you did, something someone said, or a happy thought you had, write down anything that made you feel good inside. That way you can end your day with a happy thought and set yourself up for a night of sweet dreams and a good tomorrow.

Once you've logged a few months of these happy moments, it's so fun to look back at your bright spots. Often, they can be little instances that you may have forgotten had you not written them down, and it's heartwarming to reflect on them. Plus, you'll always have them to look back on to help break you out of a funk!

(10) **JOURNAL YOUR RESPONSE:** *What healthy living can do for me.* Remember those healthy things you love from 10-Minute Fix no. 1? Now it's time to get to writing about how they're helping you out. For this journaling topic, we want you to write about how working health and fitness into your life is making a difference for you. What areas of your life are they improving? How have they benefited you already? How do you anticipate they will benefit you in the future? Has healthy living introduced you to new people or new fun activities? Has it decreased your need for unhealthy vices? Are you making yourself a priority as you never have before? Look at all of the different areas of your life and see how your new healthy lifestyle has benefited them, from your work, to your play, to your relationships. Once you're done writing, spend a minute or two thinking about the far-reaching impact of your healthy habits. Are you surprised at the effects they've had all around?

CHAPTER 6

Get Out of Your Comfort Zone

....

If your previous attempts at healthier living had you bored to tears, we have to break it to you: you were doing it wrong! Living well should *never* be boring. Being an FBG is all about putting the fun in fitness and having a sense of adventure when it comes to living a healthy lifestyle. If you've done the same old workouts in the same old order followed by the same old post-workout recovery snack . . . well, it's no wonder you've grown a little itchy from time to time and gotten off track. Bland is boring and variety is the spice of life, especially when it comes to workouts and healthy eats.

So how do you keep the fun and interest in healthy living? The trick is to get out of your comfort zone. You try workouts that might be totally new for you—ones you think you might not even like. You sample new foods that will keep your belly full and make you happy. You set small goals to push yourself to achieve bigger goals and meet new accomplishments.

Not only does trying new routines and switching things in your workout do wonders for your mindset, but banishing workout boredom also keeps your body guessing. And when you keep your body guessing, you keep seeing awesome progress in your fitness. You just keep getting better and better.

Sure, when you try new recipes or new exercise classes, not every one of them will be a hit. But if you don't try them, you'll never find that new healthy favorite dish or that new workout class that you adore. Even if something doesn't come naturally to you the first time, that doesn't mean you're bad at it or that it's not worth doing again; sometimes the greatest rewards come when you've had to work hard. Pushing yourself to try new things and attain new highs opens new doors to the world.

This mindset works for your whole life, too, not just your health. Really getting out and living life—facing your fears along the way, and making new discoveries—can help you out in other areas of your life, like your career, your relationships, and just about everything. In this chapter, we give you the tools to get and stay motivated, overcome obstacles, set goals, and obliterate plateaus. Are you ready to get out of your comfort zone? It's not as uncomfortable as you might think!

Embracing the Healthy Journey

You've probably seen the motivational poster: "It's not the destination, it's the journey." As cliché as that might be, it's *so* true when it comes to being an FBG. Because being healthy *is* all about the journey. It's not about finding the fastest or easiest path to the finish line because, well, there is no finish line. Once you're fit, you have to stay fit. Once you've lost weight, you have to maintain that success. It's not a train you get on and then get off. But don't be overwhelmed by that; our plan is to help you love it so it doesn't have a stop and start. You don't want to go on a diet; you want to keep living the full, energized, happy life.

Don't get down about the thought that you're never done or that you're never "finished." What would you do when you've lost the weight or met that fitness goal? Do you give up all the awesomeness you've added to your life? That's too sad to consider!

When you embrace the FBG lifestyle, you're also embracing the idea of a constantly evolving you. Don't be hard on yourself because you're not where you want to be; just look at any weaker areas as places to improve. If there is something specific you don't like, use that knowledge to create a new goal so that you really push yourself to make a change. You're gaining knowledge and confidence about living a fun, healthy life and learning why that's what you want to be doing. You should always be setting new goals, making new plans, trying new things. Don't think of it as a marathon that never ends; think of it as a marathon with tons of awesome scenery and detours and obstacle courses and rest stops along the way to making you the best FBG you can be.

Setting Smart Goals

Goal-setting is a huge part of being an FBG. Goals give us direction and purpose in our workouts and life. If you're like us and love making checklists, specific goals can be especially fun to set so that you can enjoy achieving them and crossing them off your list! Goals make you push yourself to be the best you can be and often help you achieve accomplishments you never thought possible. But you can't just fling a goal into the universe and will it to happen. You have to be smart about it. Really S.M.A.R.T.!

SMART goals are goals that are specific, measurable, attainable, realistic, and timely. That's a fancy way of saying that they'll help you organize your thoughts, clarify your ambitions, and create a clear plan on how to achieve them. Set them the right way, and you'll establish a pattern for setting and achieving goals that will always have you building on success, and you'll never be left feeling as if you've gotten in over your head. What does that look like in the real world? Let us paint a picture for you with words.

Specific: Getting specific about a goal gives you a precise point to aim for; it'll put you on a trajectory for success before you even begin. Get as precise as you can in goal setting: What do you want to do? How will you achieve it? Why do you want to do it? Who will be involved? Will you need a personal trainer? A running buddy? A babysitter for the kids?

Measurable: Goals such as "lose inches" or "work out more" are great *ideas*, but as goals they're pretty flimsy. Why? Because it's too hard to know if you succeeded. To have a truly SMART goal, you need to be able to assign a number to it—a way to *measure* your success. If you want to lose inches, how many? If you want to work out more, for how many minutes a week?

Attainable: When setting goals, you should feel a little bit like Goldilocks: they shouldn't be too hard, or too easy—they should be just right. You want to challenge yourself, but not so much that you get frustrated and give up. You want them to be manageable, but not so manageable that you can achieve them without any thought or effort. So give yourself a challenge, but don't bite off more than you can chew. Maybe getting into the Olympics in a sprint event isn't possible, but you could definitely shave a few seconds off of your fastest mile. Maybe as a running newbie a marathon is slightly out of reach, but you could sign up for your first 5K. Your goals should be challenging enough that you feel a sense of pride when you achieve them, and not so challenging that you're totally miserable as you work toward them.

Realistic: Make sure your goal is realistic for you and your lifestyle. Is it something you truly want to do? Is it something you can reasonably work toward? Do you have the time to take the steps to make it happen? Take a marathon, for example. It's not just about being able to run for several hours straight on race day; it's hours and hours of training each week leading up to the race. How much of your lifestyle will have to change in order to fit that amount of work in? Are you going to be willing and able to make those changes? If a goal seems unrealistic to your life, bring it down a step until you can truthfully commit to it.

Timely: With an open-ended goal, it can be easy to procrastinate. But if you set a specific date or timeline, you're much more likely to kick it into gear and go. So whether it's a date a month or two in the future or a specific span of weeks or months, set a time stamp on your goal.

Here are a few examples of SMART goals vs. not-so-SMART goals.

Not so smart: Eat more veggies.
SMART: Eat at least five servings of fruits and veggies, at least five days of the week for the next month.

FROM THE FBGs
Biggest Fitness Accomplishment

FROM ERIN: I've never considered myself a runner. Sure, I've dabbled here and there, but I've never been one to sign up for races, and I've certainly never fallen in love with the sport. So when Jenn and a couple other FBGs decided we should all sign up for a 10K (6.2 miles), I was a little nervous. I had a couple of months to train, but I was scared of injury and six miles of misery, as well as having to walk the whole race because I'd bitten off more than I could chew.

Training for the race wasn't awesome. I'd get interrupted 10 minutes into a treadmill training run at the gym by the gym daycare calling me back for one of my crying kiddos. My knee started hurting a couple of weeks in, and I had to take an almost two-week break until I could run on it again. But I kept with it; I ran when I could and I felt moderately prepared by race day.

When race day hit, the girls and I were pumped up. I'd driven into Brooklyn from New Jersey, parked in a parking spot fit for a ladybug, and I felt like I could do anything. Even though it was freezing before the race, I had so much nervous energy and I was ready to run. So I did. And not only did I finish, but I finished strong, feeling good.

A 10K might not seem like a big deal to a seasoned runner. But for me, hitting that mileage was a *big* deal. It didn't make me want to run a marathon or anything (the thought makes me shudder, frankly), but it did open my eyes to the fact that I can do more than I give myself credit for. That pushing myself to do something I'd never done before was a worthwhile goal. I ran a 10K, and no one can take that away from me.

Not so smart: Run my first 5K!
SMART: Build up to running at least 30 minutes straight by jogging/walking for 30 minutes, three times a week, by the end of May.

Not so smart: Run faster.
SMART: Take one minute off my personal 5K record at the race in May by adding sprint intervals twice a week to my training plan.

Remember, your goals are for you, so set the ones that will get you excited to achieve them. Once you meet a goal, set the bar a little higher and start on the next one. And if you don't meet your goal? Go back over the SMART criteria and make some adjustments. And don't get down; use it as motivation to really give you something to work toward.

Baby-Step It to the Finish

We know that it's tempting to want to set huge goals when you start something and are all jazzed up about it, but if you've tried to pick up healthy habits that haven't stuck in the past, it may be because you have bitten off more than you could chew. And while we love the idea of setting fantastic, ambitious goals, beware of the burnout and injuries that can come from aiming too high, too fast.

Success builds on success, and chunking goals into smaller, manageable pieces helps you succeed—which in turn gives you more confidence and spunk and determination to do even more. Taking baby steps to achieve your goals helps ease you into what can be intimidating; it helps you slowly creep out of your comfort zone without being too uncomfortable. Eventually, you'll look back and be amazed at what you've accomplished—and just how far you've come with those baby steps!

If you have weight to lose, you might be overwhelmed by the thought of what seems like 50 impossible pounds. But making a goal to lose 4 pounds in a month seems totally attainable. In our experience, when it comes to weight loss, breaking down goals into smaller, more manageable targets, like losing 1 to 2 pounds per week, can lead to more success. With smaller goals, you can celebrate each mini success before focusing on the next few pounds—and avoid getting distracted or down on yourself when progress slows.

It's okay to have a big, ambitious goal in the back of your mind that you want to achieve; in fact, that's wonderful. But the best way to make it a reality is to break it down into the baby steps you'll have to take to get there. There's a fine line between pushing yourself hard and pushing yourself too hard, and you have to be aware enough of your abilities and weaknesses to know the difference. Looking at your long-term goals and dividing them into reasonable short-term goals can give you the building blocks you need to achieve them!

Rewards Rock

Setting rewards that complement your SMART goals is the perfect way to keep motivated and on track. Rewards give you something to look forward to and can be a fantastic way to celebrate your progress. Plus, rewards just make you feel good! So it makes total sense that they're part of the FBG lifestyle.

Getting out of your comfort zone and setting new, big goals can

REWARDS ON A BUDGET

Rewards don't *have* to be pricey items. Even little things here and there can get you psyched to keep on with your healthy choices. Here are a few ideas for all kinds of budgets!

Free
- Spend quiet time reading at the library.
- Watch your favorite guilty-pleasure TV show.
- Take a nap.
- Go for a walk through a beautiful park.
- Have a day where your only goal is to do what makes you happy.

$10 or Less
- Buy a new fun nail polish color to paint your nails.
- Purchase a magazine or gently used book.
- Get a new pair of undies or socks.
- Go to a local museum.
- Have coffee with a friend.

$30 or Less
- Buy a new workout DVD.
- Go out for a glass of wine with a friend and pick up the tab.
- Get a manicure or pedicure.
- Hit the clearance rack of your favorite clothing or activewear store.
- Pick out a new fun accessory like sunglasses, earrings, or a scarf.

$50 or Less
- Treat yourself and a friend to a class at that hot new workout studio.
- Cook yourself a homemade steak dinner with a nice salad and roasted veggies.

- Go ahead and buy that pricey bottle of champagne or wine.
- Donate to your favorite charity.
- Buy a new sports bra that fits perfectly.

$100 or Less
- Book a massage.
- Go out on the town for a fancy dinner.
- Get a new pair of workout shoes.
- Attend a concert, play, or other performance.
- Find the perfect little black dress that makes you feel fantastic.

While a lot of fitness professionals will tell you to always set nonfood rewards, we actually like having some food-related ones in there. Harkening back to our discussion of balance, food is something to be enjoyed, not restricted. We believe that splurging on higher-quality eats and drinks than usual can be a fabulous way to celebrate your progress—and a way to work special treats into your life. As we always say, all good things in moderation!

Remember, small and steady wins the race; and goals and rewards along the way just make it all that much more fun. So enjoy setting goals, reaching them, and celebrating your progress week after week, month after month, and year after year!

seem overwhelming, but giving yourself little reward pick-me-ups along the way can make the entire process easier and more enjoyable. The key is to pick rewards that matter to you and get you excited—and then match them appropriately to your goals. Smaller goals, like those that take a month or less to achieve (such as adding an extra serving of veggies to your day or setting out to stretch after every workout), should have smaller rewards (like splurging on a few flowers for yourself or downloading a new song for your workout playlist). Then the big long-term goals, like training for a 10K or losing twenty pounds, get bigger, more substantial rewards (like a full day at the spa, or a weekend getaway, or money to spend on a new wardrobe that fits).

Setting rewards isn't an exact science, but having a goal—large or small—to reach every two to four weeks is ideal for keeping the rewards infrequent enough to make them meaningful but often enough that they work.

Six Common Setbacks and How to Overcome Them

If the whole idea of healthy living feels so far out of your comfort zone that you don't know where to begin, we're here to help. We've been around the fitness block a time or two, and along the way we've identified a few setbacks that seem to trip people up—and solutions to overcome them.

1. **TIME.** Have you ever heard anyone say she is looking for ways to fill up her overabundance of spare time? From work, to relationships, to kids, to keeping the house clean, it can feel as if there is not a sliver of time to use for workouts or making healthy meals. But we'll let you in on a little secret: it's not really about the time. It's about making the time a priority.

   How to overcome: We all have the same number of hours in a day. Instead of repeating the "I don't have time" mantra, tell yourself, "I make time to take care of me because it's important." Say it often enough and it'll be your new reality.

Also, start rethinking what you consider a "workout." Embrace mini bouts of exercise and try to fit more of them into your days—they really do add up. If you still struggle to find even 10 minutes in your day to get your body moving, it's time to multitask. Turn TV time into toning time. Park farther away from the store. Turn business meetings into walking meetings, pace the office, or do squats during conference calls. Play time with your kids can turn into strength and cardio if you can head to the playground and add in some push-ups and squats. And healthy eating? It takes no more time than anything else once you stock up on the right basics.

2. **MONEY.** While you certainly can spend a fortune on the latest equipment, clothing, shoes, heart rate monitors, and gym memberships, being *sans* funds is no excuse for not being the fittest you that you can be. In fact, the best piece of fitness equipment in the world is your body—and you can do every side of the FBG Fitness Triangle with nothing more than some comfy clothes and your sneakers.

How to overcome: There are loads of free or nearly free activities you can do that require only supportive shoes, like walking, running, stretching, and doing body-weight exercises like push-ups, lunges, and crunches. For a small cost, you can add in activities like jumping rope, shooting hoops, playing tennis, dancing in your living room, or throwing a football with a pal. Head to the Internet to find free workouts and videos you can do at home with little to no equipment—there are thousands out there.

Likewise, eating healthy doesn't have to be expensive. And if you're preparing your meals at home, you'll have delicious options that are easily available all the time. Simply make it a priority to cook at home most of the time; eating out is way more costly than cooking yourself. Pack your lunches and snacks so you're not tempted to hit the work cafeteria or head to the local drive-thru. Make large batches of your favorite healthy meals so that you can use leftovers for lunches.

3. **PERFECTIONISM.** Almost all of us have made resolutions that we are sure we are going to stick with, only to have them fall apart in a couple of weeks. We turn over that new leaf, determined to get on a healthy eating plan and exercise every day. We plan the perfect schedule and plan the perfect healthy menu for the week. The first week goes great. But the second week, we miss a workout because we got a flat tire. And then we have a piece of chocolate cake at a co-worker's birthday party. Two slipups, so our diet is toast, right? Wrong! So, so wrong. The illusion of perfection can be a huge hang-up for even the most practical people. Because living this lifestyle isn't an all-or-nothing approach—it's the anti-diet, remember?

How to overcome: When your goal is perfection all the time, you're just setting yourself up for failure. One of the big aspects of living the FBG life is that your lifestyle has to be realistic. Is it realistic to *never* have a piece of cake? No. Is it realistic to work out *every* day? No. Life happens. Workouts get skipped and treats are had. And, yes, sometimes one piece of cake leads to another. It's not the end of the world! Having an all-or-nothing mindset is a slippery slope; because you never cut yourself a break or allow yourself any wiggle room, when life's slipups happen you keep sliding down that slope. Instead, you have to get right back on that horse. Don't just put off your healthy lifestyle until tomorrow; make each meal count. Overeat at breakfast? Lunch is a whole new meal for you to make choices that will be filling and nutritious. Snack too much mid-afternoon? Make your dinner as healthy as possible. Don't see splurges as setbacks; use them in your 80/20 plan for awesome results and you won't feel deprived.

4. **LOSS OF MOTIVATION.** The first few weeks of your FBG journey, you were on fire! Unstoppable and rocking small changes. But as the weeks have ticked by, you've slipped here or "forgotten" there. And now, well, your motivation to work out and eat right is gone, baby, gone. Going for a jog sounds like torture; and when you do get to the gym, the elliptical just isn't as much fun as it used to be. Not to mention that you seriously can't bear the thought of eating another grilled chicken breast.

   How to overcome: Motivation wanes for everyone (even us!) from time to time, so the key is to not beat yourself up about it. Instead, do

ENERGIZE!
Look the Part

We're no strangers to wearing our grubbiest shorts and our rattiest T-shirts to exercise. After all, you don't need to have expensive, fancy clothing to get an effective workout. But there's no denying that when you look good, you feel good—and when your workout clothes rock, it can take your workout to a rockin' new level. So next time you're just not in the mood to get off the couch, put on the prettiest workout clothes you've got that make you feel like your sexiest workout self. (And if you've got nothing you love, new workout duds can be a great reward for a goal well met!) Dress the part of an energized FBG and soon you'll be acting the part, too!

something about it—and fast. Get reacquainted with not just why you want to lose weight but also why you *deserve* to lose the weight and be your healthiest right now. Go back and read through some of your previous journaling exercises. Get back in touch with your Superhero Alter Ego. If you're really in a rut, you may need a big ol' change, like setting entirely new goals, or swapping your indoor workouts for outdoor ones, or changing your cardio goals for strength goals. If you're just a little unmotivated, it might just take a fun new recipe or trying a new type of group exercise class to bust you through. No matter how much you need to get your healthy living mojo back, hold your head up high, tell yourself you're a fit and motivated person, and then go out and do the darn thing, making a point to change things up. Boredom be gone!

5. **OBSESSIVE THOUGHTS.** You know that *diet* is a four-letter word and you've broken up with the scale. But you still can't seem to stop thinking about what you ate, what you will eat, and how in the world you'll burn off that extra slice of pizza you didn't need last night but ate anyway. And are these pants really fitting better or did they just stretch out? Although we've been working hard to get a more positive and healthy mindset in your head, the obsessive thoughts and tendencies many of us have had since we were teens about weight are sometimes the hardest to overcome. They just keep creeping up! So we fall back into old patterns, and we obsess. We start ignoring our true hunger signs and we overdo it at the gym. And then we're, oh my God, so *hungry*. So we overeat, and the whole obsessive process starts again. Ugh!

   How to overcome: If you start to retreat to unhealthy obsessive patterns, the first step is awareness. Become cognizant of any obsessive thoughts you're having. Then—without judging that thought—ask yourself: "What kind of thoughts would an FBG have about this? Would she be worried about not burning enough calories today or if she looked like she had a muffin top in that tank?" The answer you'll get will most likely be "No, she'd be looking forward to the new yoga DVD she's trying later that afternoon and wearing clothes that made her feel good." The more you can objectively look at your thoughts and make a little space so that you can see if they're really serving your goals and healthy life or not, the better.

Whenever you get into an obsessive or nonloving thought about yourself, try to redirect that thinking. Pretend that those not-so-healthy thoughts are like a bad TV show you're watching. Instead of sitting and listening to them, change the dial to something more uplifting and positive, like thinking of things in your life that you're grateful for and reliving a time when you accomplished one of your goals. And if even after doing all of this, you still can't seem to break the obsessive pattern, go back to Chapters 1 and 5. Those 10-Minute Fixes will definitely help!

6. PLAYING THE VICTIM. You've been doing everything, quite literally, by the book. You eat like an FBG, think like an FBG, and work out like an FBG. But while you are feeling better, you're just not getting the results you want. No, scratch that, you're getting results, but not as fast as you want them. You feel frustrated and often ask yourself, *Why won't this stupid weight just come off? Why is losing weight so hard for me?!*

How to overcome: We all want fast results. But the magic bullet for weight loss doesn't exist. It takes time. Just like you didn't gain all of your weight overnight, you can't expect to lose it overnight, either. This can be a tough pill to swallow (not many of us like to fess up about our own shortcomings!), but you have to take responsibility for the actions that got you to this point. Change is always possible, even if it isn't always easy. So if you start to get impatient and play the "Why Me?" game, get real with yourself about your situation and consider why a quick fix is not the answer nor will it ever be the answer. Head back to Chapter 5 to get in touch with your attitude of gratitude and then repeat this phrase until you don't just feel it, but you *know* it to be true: *I am strong. I am beautiful. I am worthy.*

It may not seem like this will do much, but by being grateful and saying this simple affirmation over and over, your mindset will change from that of a victim to that of an empowered woman who has the confidence and self-respect to fully care for herself. And this is the essence of being a Fit Bottomed Girl for life!

Also, don't lose sight of all of the amazing things that *are* happening. You should be seeing all kinds of benefits: more energy, healthier skin, shinier hair, stronger muscles, a willingness to try new things, a more positive outlook! These are all things that the scale can't detect but should make you feel really, really good and accomplished. Setbacks happen to the best of us, but don't let them get you down. The best part about being an FBG is continuing on, picking yourself up and dusting yourself off, getting back on that horse, and treating every day as an opportunity to be your best self.

Getting out of your comfort zone   be it by set
ting new goals, coming up with new rewards, or
breaking through your own mental barriers—doesn't have to
take tons of time. Try these 10-Minute Fixes to get you busting
through plateaus and reaching your fit and healthy dreams!

(1) **SET GOALS FOR ALL AREAS OF YOUR LIFE.** Goal-setting might
seem a bit intimidating at first. *Where do I start? What do I want
to do? Which goal should I focus on first?* But don't feel lost. We
have a simple process for getting you to figure out your long-
term and short-term goals. Here's how to create goals to bust out
of your comfort zone.

Pick an area of focus: Being an FBG is definitely about eating
right and moving your body. But it's also about being healthy
in other areas of your life, such as your career and your
relationships. That's why it makes sense to pick the key areas
you'd like to address with your goals. We've found that it's best
to not go after more than two big goals at a time. Begin by
figuring out which areas your goals are going to home in on:
fitness, nutrition, balance, career, or relationships?

Tap into your desires: Ask yourself this of each area: What have
I always wanted to do in this area but haven't? Is it running a
5K, 10K, or a half or full marathon? Going vegan? Walking the
Great Wall of China or hiking the Appalachian Trail? Making a
career switch? Renewing your wedding vows? If the answers
to this question give you excited/nervous butterflies, you're
definitely on the right path to finding some things that push
you out of your comfort zone!

Get SMART: Take the list you just brainstormed and see which one from each area sets itself up best as a specific-measurable-attainable-realistic-and-timely (SMART) goal. That's going to be your goal!

Set a plan to get there: You have your goal, so now it's time to set the timeline for when you'd like to reach it and how you'll measure your progress. As previously discussed, be sure to "chunk" your large goal down into smaller goals to aim for as you go.

Reward yo'self: Choose the awesome rewards to go with your short-term and long-term goals. Pick ones that you'll really look forward to!

Do the dang thing: Enjoy the whole process of reaching your healthy dreams, be it weight loss, running a race, or even getting that big promotion you've been wanting!

(2) **TAKE THE MINI-GOAL CHALLENGE.** We've been focusing on long-term and short-term goals—and many of them are centered on events or doing certain things in your life. But as long as they meet that SMART criteria, goals don't have to be one-size-fits-all. In fact, we encourage you to get creative and invent goals that are fun, meaningful to you, and fit into your daily life. To get you thinking outside of the box, try incorporating these sample mini-minute goals. Then brainstorm your own fun ones once you've conquered these!

No negative thoughts for 10 minutes: Do you talk to yourself like you're your own best friend? Make a goal to banish the Negative Nancy in your head for a full 10 minutes by becoming aware of those thoughts and focusing on the positive. Don't worry if it takes you a while to build up to 10 minutes—just start with how long you can go without a negative thought about yourself and then build from there. And as your positive mental power gets stronger, expand this goal to 20, 30, 40, and more minutes. Heck, eventually we'd love to have you giving yourself self-love all day, every day!

Move for 10 minutes nonstop: Can't fit a "formal" workout into your day? Set a goal to move for 10 minutes nonstop. It doesn't matter if you're doing laundry, chasing after your kids, or even pacing around your office; set a goal to move your body for 10 minutes without stopping. This is an easy goal you can challenge yourself to do each and every day!

Take a minute every hour of the day for you: Incorporate more "me time" into your life by not just challenging yourself to set aside 10 minutes a day just for you but also by setting a goal to take one minute that's just for you every hour for 10 hours. Set a reminder or alert on your computer or your phone that buzzes on the hour, and then do something that feels good to you. Go to your favorite website, do a few jumping jacks, refill your water bottle, take some deep breaths, pet your dog, do your favorite yoga pose, just sit and look out the window—it doesn't matter as long as it leaves you feeling good!

(3) **SET UP A REWARDS JAR.** We've already given you lots of fun ideas for rewards, but one that almost everyone adores? The rewards jar. Simply take a container that you're not using (even a shoe box, piggy bank, or gift bag you've been saving to reuse), and every time you work out or make a healthier choice (like

10-Minute Fixes

swapping your diet soda order for water or calling a friend to emote instead of hitting the fridge for "support") put a little bit of money in the jar. It can be a quarter, a dollar, $5—whatever works best for you. Then, after a set period of time (we recommend at least a week or two), count up your earnings and use it to do something or buy something you'd like to reward yourself with. Feel free to really "pretty up" your rewards jar, too, with stickers (hey, you're never too old for them!), images from magazines that you've cut out, or by writing little inspirational sayings on it.

We love how this idea is so simple yet gives such concrete results. Not only is it a good way to "save" money for your rewards but it also allows you to see just how many good choices you're making!

(4) **SEE YOUR SUCCESS.** Say you've picked a huge goal—one that kind of, okay mostly, scares the ever-loving heck out of you, like doing a triathlon or setting out to cook a healthy dinner for your super-foodie boss. Yes, you're excited for it, but it just seems so . . . *big*. And, again, scary! In addition to chunking your huge goals into smaller, more attainable ones, taking 10 minutes to visualize yourself doing the impossible is a fantastic way to turn that dream into the possible—and face your fears head-on along the way.

The next time you're doing steady-state cardio, like running, walking, or stepping it out on the StairMaster (you'll want to be indoors for this, as you'll be kind of zoning out and don't want to worry about tripping or cars or other safety risks like that!), take 10 minutes of your workout to see yourself reaching your goals.

Visualize crossing that finish line, or feeling comfortable and confident in that swimsuit, or happily choosing healthy foods even with your biggest trigger foods around you. In that goal-reaching moment, how do you feel? What sounds do you hear? What sensations are going on in your body? How are you breathing? What emotions are you feeling? Are there any special smells? Tie in to all five of your senses to really get the full experience.

Ten minutes may seem like a long time to do this, but we want you to get super-familiar with the image of yourself reaching your goals. Professional athletes and Olympians have long been using visualizations as part of their training to mentally prepare themselves for competition and stay motivated. And we think if it's good enough for the pros, it's good enough for you! Truth is, when you can see yourself doing something, you're more likely to do it. So we say see it, and see it often!

FIT BOTTOMED MANTRA

"If you can dream it, you can do it."
—WALT DISNEY

(5) **CALL B.S. ON YOURSELF.** Excuses are just that—*excuses*. They're little white lies we use (or straight up come up with) to help us justify a behavior. They are things within our control that we twist ever so slightly to seem as though we couldn't influence the outcome. But we know deep down that we could.

The opposite of excuses are reasons. These are bona fide situations that make a healthy choice or workout impossible. Stuff like "I got a flat tire and missed Zumba," or "I got snowed in and couldn't get out to buy fresh produce," or "I have the flu and can't move, let alone get off the couch." These are not the-dog-ate-my-homework kinds of events; these are reasons. Things out of your control.

So take a few minutes and look at your routine and your life. Where and when are you saying you have a reason to do or not do something? Now ask yourself: *Is it really a reason? Or is it an excuse?* Believe us, your gut will know the answer; you just have to be open enough to accept and embrace the truth. Remember, no one is perfect—and we *all* do this!

For any "reasons" you have, cut yourself some slack. They're legit. For any "excuses," make a plan to bust them down into healthier, more empowered decisions. Tell a supportive loved one about your excuse *du jour* and how you're making a pact with yourself (and him or her) to no longer let it hold you back. Then set up some kind of regular visual reminder that says "No excuses" in a place that you'll see at least a few times a day. You can set up an auto-reminder on your phone or computer, or you can leave yourself notes on your mirror, in your closet, on your fridge, and on your desk. Design these in any way you want, but when you look at them, don't see them as some kind of personal punishment. Instead, use them as motivation to be your absolute best. In fact, seeing them should ignite an inner fire in you to reach your goals—no excuses!

(6) **BUST THROUGH A PLATEAU.** Whether it's in regard to losing weight or getting fit, plateaus happen to the best of us. And we know from experience that there's nothing more frustrating than

having your progress come to a screeching halt. What's important to understand, though, is that plateaus can happen for a variety of reasons—some of which have to do with healthy eating and workouts and some of which don't. So take 10 minutes to answer these five questions to see what sneaky things might be getting you stuck—and then learn how to get unstuck!

HOW MANY HOURS OF SLEEP ARE YOU GETTING A NIGHT?

Plateau Buster: Aim for 7 to 9 hours each night. If you're regularly sleeping less than seven hours a night, sleep deprivation may be slowing your progress. Not getting enough sleep at night has been linked to weight gain, increased hunger, and slower recovery from workouts. Not to mention that you just feel too tired to do much of anything when you're not getting your zzz's!

HOW MANY OFF DAYS ARE YOU TAKING FROM WORKOUTS?

Plateau Buster: Aim for 1 to 2 days a week. You can totally get too much of a good thing, which is why it's essential to give your body at least one day a week of rest. When you don't give your body enough time to recover, it stresses your system, which can lead to—you guessed it—the stoppage of results and possibly even overuse injuries. This is why it's also important to try not to do the same exact type of workout on back-to-back days so that your body fully has time to recover.

WHEN'S THE LAST TIME YOU SWITCHED UP YOUR WORKOUTS?

Plateau Buster: Change your workouts every four to six weeks.
The really cool thing about your body is that it adapts—and gets better and more efficient the longer you do something. So the workout you started three months ago? It's not nearly as hard now as the first time you did it. The not-so-cool part of your adaptability, though, is that you have to regularly switch things up to keep your body challenged. That means that every month or so you must change either the frequency (how many workouts you do a week), intensity (how hard you're working), the type of workout you're doing, or the amount of time you're doing a particular activity. Switching things up not only keeps plateaus at bay but it also keeps things fresh so that your motivation doesn't plateau, either!

ARE YOU BEING MINDFUL WHEN YOU EAT?

Plateau Buster: Eat without any distractions. You may think you're eating the right amount—not too much and not too little—but if you're not fully aware of what you're noshing, you might be eating more or less than you think. Both over- and undereating can lead to plateaus (overeating because it causes an excess of energy, which gets stored as fat, and undereating because it puts your body in a state of starvation and slows your metabolism, making it harder to lose weight). So be sure to check in with your hunger and fullness levels each time you eat. Also, minimize distractions when eating—no TV, no work, no multitasking. Sit down for every meal and snack, put them on a plate, and be mindful and aware of each tasty bite!

ARE YOU OVERLY STRESSED?

Plateau Buster: Develop a relaxation habit. Chronic stress—the kind you face every day and seem to never get a break from—has all kinds of negative effects, including weight gain, poor quality of sleep, headaches, and depression, making it more likely that a tough workout will leave you feeling sore and tired for longer than normal. We present loads of stress-busting strategies in the next chapter, but for now begin setting aside a few minutes a day to chill it on out. From a few simple deep breaths to meditation to a few yoga poses, a little downtime can be just what you need to overcome that plateau.

It may be possible that you have more than one of these things interfering with your progress. If that's the case, don't freak! Just pick one area to focus on making a little more FBG-friendly. Once you've got the Plateau Buster in place and you're feeling good, tackle another one.

And, please, have some patience with your body. It's a complex creation and one that doesn't always show change on the outside as quickly as we'd like. But that doesn't mean that amazing things aren't happening. So give it some love, take care of it, and trust the FBG process!

(7) **PUSH-YOURSELF WORKOUTS.** Working outside of your comfort zone—either by doing activities or moves you're not used to or

working at an intensity that physically feels uncomfortable—is a surefire way to get fitter and see just how much your body can do. In order to take your fitness to the next level, try one of these three workouts. Don't worry if they feel awkward at first; the whole point is to learn something new!

CARDIO WORKOUT: STRIDERS

Doing striders, which is simply a common drill used by runners to increase pace and get used to running at faster speeds, is an amazing HIIT workout that boosts fitness and will take you to the next level. Try this one on a treadmill, a track, a path, or a trail, and get ready to push yourself outside of your comfort zone; this is definitely advanced!

Warm-up: Walk for 2 minutes.
Striders interval: Walk quickly or jog at a regular pace for 30 steps (left/right equals one step). Then increase your pace for another 20 steps. Then run fast or sprint for 10 steps. Repeat the striders interval series for 6 minutes.
Cool-down: Walk for 2 minutes.

STRENGTH WORKOUT: FUN WITH A MEDICINE BALL

Weighted medicine balls are a great tool and can totally take your workouts up a notch, because they force your body to move in extremely functional ways that mimic your everyday life—just with more weight and more of a balance element. Almost all gyms have these, or you can buy them at a local sporting goods store. Beginners, try a 4- to 6-pound weighted ball; intermediate and advanced, grab an 8- to 12-pound ball.

Warm-up: Lightly jog for 2 minutes.

Medicine ball series: Do the below circuit as many times as you can in 6 minutes. (And it's totally A-okay if you can only get through this once!)

- **5 medicine ball push-ups:** Place both hands on the medicine ball, with your hands balanced on the ball and your fingers and thumbs touching so that you make a diamond shape, and lower down into a push-up with your arms close to your body. Feel free to be down on your knees or up on your toes.

- **5 rock and rolls:** From a sit-up position with your knees bent and the medicine ball in your hands above your head, use your momentum to move your hands and medicine ball out in front of your chest and roll yourself up and into a standing position with your arms extended out in front of you.

- **5 wall throws:** First, find a wall that you can throw a heavy ball against. Once found, stand about 6 feet from the wall and take the ball in your hands and throw it out at the wall like you're passing a basketball to someone. As it bounces back off the wall, catch it. Be careful to not clock yourself in the face, obviously.

Cool-down: Walk for 2 minutes.

FLEXIBILITY WORKOUT: STABILITY BALL STRETCH

Get ready to stretch out of your comfort zone with this feel-good flexibility workout that uses a large stability ball!

- **5 ball breaths:** Standing and holding the ball in your hands, squat down and then stand up as you take a deep breath and raise the ball overhead. As you lift and lower, think about really standing tall and elongating the body, and breathe out. Continue flowing and pairing the movement to your breath.

- **Hip circles:** Sit on the ball nice and tall. Now slowly circle your hips around for 30 seconds in one direction, really focusing on getting as wide of a circle as possible. Then reverse the direction for another 30 seconds. Go slowly enough that you're not worried about falling off!

- **Back stretch:** Sitting on the ball, roll down so that the ball is supporting the natural curve of your back and your knees are bent. Roll back as far as is comfortable, straightening the knees, as you feel the amazing back stretch! Enjoy for a full minute.

- **Chest stretch:** From a back stretch position, roll down a little more so that your knees are deeply bent. Extend your arms out to the side and then back, and lean from one side to the other, holding for 30 seconds on each side.

- **One-handed child's pose:** Get in an all-fours position with the stability ball in front of you. Place one hand on the stability ball while you sit back on your heels. Hold for 30 seconds while you feel a stretch down one side of your body. Switch the ball to the other hand and repeat on that side for another 30 seconds.

- **Total body stretch:** From a standing position with the ball a couple of feet out in front of you, fold down into a forward bend. Reach out for the ball to increase the stretch in your hamstrings and lower back. Hold for a full minute.

- **5 ball breaths:** End your workout with five more of these feel-good moves.

8 **DOCUMENT YOUR HEALTHY JOURNEY.** As we keep saying, this whole healthy living thing shouldn't feel like work; it should feel like an adventure! And sometimes adventures are scary—and require documentation of your brave pursuits. So just as you would make a photo album or scrapbook for an amazing trip, we want you to create a memory book that really honors and celebrates your journey and your progress—like a souvenir book of your greatest obstacles overcome. So go out and buy a scrapbook (or make your own by using a three-ring binder with plastic sheet protectors and fun construction paper), and then spend 10 minutes gathering memories from your fit and healthy adventures for the month. Oh, and if you're not feeling crafty, consider doing this on Pinterest! Here are some fun things to include:

- **Photos:** Include plenty of personal pics, such as 5K race photos, before and after photos of weight loss, shots of your latest healthy smoothie, or softball tournament pics—anything active and healthy goes!

- **Aha moments:** Did you recently have a breakthrough when journaling? Or did you see an article in a magazine that really inspired you? Include it!

- **Health markers:** Anytime you go to the doctor, add your stats to your book. Not only is it a good way to track your cholesterol and blood pressure numbers over time, but it's plain amazing to see how your insides are changing, too!

- **Fit swag:** Not sure what to do with that race certificate or that shoelace tag? Add it to your memory book!

- **Recipes:** Created a new recipe you love? Write it out, date it, and document that healthy creation!

Then, every month or so, take another 10 minutes to add to your memory book. Over time you'll not just have a record of your healthy journey, you'll also have a whole binder of your greatest triumphs to look back on and be inspired by!

(9) **CELEBRATE YOUR SUCCESSES.** We've already discussed how amazing rewards can be at keeping you motivated and on track, but sometimes when you've done something really, *really* amazing, you need a little more than just a reward to mark the healthy occasion. You need a full-out celebration for busting out of that comfort zone! And here are four fun 10-minute ideas to do just that.

- **Plan a party:** Who says that you can't have a party to celebrate breaking up with diet soda or crossing the finish line of that half marathon? Not us! Take 10 minutes to plan out whom you'll invite, what your theme will be ("hail kale" or "born to run" are always crowd-pleasers), and what healthy snacks and drinks you'll serve. Then set a date and spread the word! (And, seriously, the idea is a bit silly, but everyone loves a party!)

• **Toast with smoothies:** Grab a few buds and your finest cocktail glasses, and then throw your favorite ingredients in the blender to whip up a tasty smoothie. Pour the smoothies into said glasses, and toast to breaking through your comfort zone!

• **Create a celebration playlist:** You can't have a celebration without good tunes! So get thee to your iPod and start creating a list of your favorite high-energy party tracks. Bonus points if you can include songs that actually have the words *celebration* and *party* in them. Then, the next time you're going for a workout, jam it on out with your celebration playlist and feel super proud of yourself!

• **Write your acceptance speech:** Always wanted to thank the academy? Here's your chance—with an FBG twist. Go ahead and grab your favorite piece of fitness equipment—a dumbbell, a pair of running shoes, your jump rope—and use it as your "award." Then go ahead: thank all those people who got you here! (And feel free to do this one with friends for fun or on your own. We know from experience that pets make fantastic audience members!)

(10) **JOURNAL YOUR RESPONSE:** *Why I want to reach my goals.* Goals are awesome, but in order to fully reach them, you have to have a reason for wanting to do so. And not just any ol' reason; you want a really strong one that comes from deep down. One that'll get you through any challenge. One that you can always tap into for motivation. Spend 10 minutes writing in your journal

172 The Fit Bottomed Girls Anti-Diet

about the reasons why you want to reach your goals. What are you working toward? What does it mean to you? How will it feel when you reach them? How will you keep your progress going? No matter your answers, keep asking yourself *why?* again and again to drill down to the deepest, most personal reasons you want to reach you goals. Once you find those deep inner reasons, you can use them as an inner flame to keep on going until you reach 'em! (And then set new goals and do it all over again!)

CHAPTER 7

Chill Out

Life is hectic. We're all busy. We're all stressed. If you're like most busy girls, you don't stop moving from the time your feet hit the floor in the morning until you get into bed at night. But if you get too busy and too frazzled, it can be easier to make excuses for skipping that workout. Grabbing the easy and often unhealthy takeout instead of cooking becomes habit rather than an exception. It's easier to fall into that negative headspace where you don't see the stress ever ending.

That's why this chapter is all about the importance of taking time out for yourself to relax and recharge. We're not just talking about taking a vacation once a year or taking off work the days the office is closed; those breaks are few and far between, and they won't do enough to help you stay balanced in your daily life. Every day, it's important to take a moment to relax and recharge. You don't have to take a long meditation weekend or schedule weekly massages to start making relaxation a priority (although you certainly can!). Simply incorporating a few moments of quiet time into and throughout your day can go a long way toward easing the stresses of daily life. Think of yourself as a battery, or a cell phone that you must plug in each night; you need that recharging to be able to work—and play—effectively the next day. Sleep is a huge part of this, but so is simple downtime.

Stop Being Over-Everythinged

Remember back in Chapter 4, when we had you practice saying no? That's because if you're a people pleaser, it can be easy to put all of your needs aside for the good of others, whether it's your friends, family, or demanding boss. But pushing yourself to the limit and putting yourself aside is a sure ticket to stress city. You get overscheduled, overworked, and overwhelmed. Doing too much for others and not enough for yourself makes you a stressed FBG!

Wondering how on earth you'll fit in time to de-stress? That's the thing: It's not about adding one more thing to your already massive to-do list. It's about making yourself a priority so that healthy living is what you're doing while you're writing that list. Living healthy will make you feel better all around—making it easier to juggle all of the balls you have in the air. You'll feel lighter, stronger, and more prepared for what life throws at you, rather than stressed and overwhelmed. Check out our tips on managing your to-dos so you can begin to carve out time to make yourself a priority again.

Compartmentalize your day. At the beginning of each week, set a few priorities that you need to get accomplished. Then make your daily to-do lists in support of each of those weekly goals. Need to

FROM THE FBGs
How to Chill It on Out

FROM JENN: I'll be the first to admit that I don't always deal with stress as well as I should. I work a lot, like intense workouts, and am used to pushing myself to the limit. I really do feel my best when I'm working toward a huge goal, like training for a race, conquering a tough move, or starting a new website or big project (or, hey, writing a book!). But, in doing so, I have a tendency to stress myself out a bit. Which is why the below activities are part of my healthy living routine!

Every day: There are two things I do each day to unwind. First, I walk my dog. Getting outside always relaxes me, and seeing my dog happy as can be, wagging her tail outside? Well, that's just pure joy. Second, I meditate. I shoot for 15 to 20 minutes when I can, but even just five minutes of sitting quietly gives my brain a much-needed break from thinking!

Every week: Once, maybe twice, a week I do a 30- to 60-minute yoga workout DVD or class, usually over the weekday lunch hour. The mix of moving, breathing, and stretching is a great way to work relaxation into my workday.

Every month: Massages might be the best things in the world. Seriously. They are Zen-inducing and an oh-so-necessary treat for my muscles and mind. They may be pricey, but I set aside the funds to get one every month; heck, just skipping a dinner or two out pays for it! For me, massages are also a great way for me to get some quiet alone time. Well, as alone as you can be with a massage therapist!

get a report written by the end of the week? Set mini-goals for each day. Want to donate the clothes you haven't worn in a year? Go through a drawer every day. House need a deep clean? Focus on a room each day. Have both a work list and a personal list so that one doesn't take precedence over the other. And most important, don't forget to include workouts and time for yourself in there!

Take breaks. It can seem counterintuitive that taking a break will actually help you get more work done, but studies have shown that brief breaks can clear your head and help you focus. After all, how often do you start to mindlessly browse the Internet because you just can't work on that report anymore? Why not get up and move around instead? A change of scenery and getting your blood pumping will give you the break you need to effectively tackle the job once you get back to it.

Put the work away. With smartphones and tablets that have the Internet and email at your fingertips 24/7, it's easy to feel the need to be available at all times. But set a time each night to put away all devices and relax. Maybe it means leaving work at the office for a night. Maybe it means checking email quickly at 7 P.M. for anything important and then turning off your devices until morning. Setting limits on your work life goes a long way to ensuring you have time for your personal pursuits. Not only that, it leaves you feeling fresher and ready to tackle the workday when you've had the opportunity to step away.

Delegate. Don't look at delegating tasks or asking for help as a sign of weakness or that you can't handle all of your responsibilities. It's actually a sign of strength to know when you need a hand and to have a great support network that can see you through the crazy times. Sure, others might not do something exactly how you do it, but does it really have to be done your exact way? The weight of the world shouldn't be on your shoulders alone, especially if you're putting most of the pressure on yourself.

Embrace imperfection. You can't do it all, and you certainly can't do it all perfectly. You don't need a perfect diet or exercise plan to be fit and healthy, so similarly, cut yourself some slack in other areas of your life, too. Strive to do your best, but don't beat yourself up when you goof. So your laundry sits in a pile for another day so you have time to hit the gym? So be it. Your house doesn't have to look like it came out of a magazine. Aim for that healthy balance we talked about before, not perfection.

Know your limits so you recognize when you're hitting your frazzled breaking point. Don't keep pushing yourself to do more, be better, and be perfect when it's affecting you and making you too stressed to enjoy life! Check out our 10-Minute Fixes for even more ways to chill, calm, and get more time for yourself.

What Stress Does to Your Bod

You probably already know that stress doesn't *feel* good. It zaps your energy, your motivation, and your lust for life. You feel run-down, tired, cranky. You feel like there is never enough time to do what you need and want to do, and so you always feel overwhelmed and like you can never catch up. Heck, you might be feeling that way right now. But besides just making you feel bad, stress can do some pretty cray-cray things to your body. From messing with your weight, to your workouts, to your cravings, to your overall health, stress is a six-letter word that acts more like a four-letter word when it gets out of hand.

Known as our "fight or flight response," our body's reaction to stress is a leftover from our cavelady days, when our bodies would kick out specific hormones to help us be alert and ready to move in scary, possibly life-threatening situations. (Sabertooth tiger . . . run!) Through various processes in the body, these hormones basically flood our bodies with energy in any way possible—suppressing the immune system, jacking with blood sugar levels, turning off our natural feelings of hunger—to get us through said emergency situation. Then, once the big stressful event is over (Sabertooth tiger crisis averted . . . hooray!), our bodies have cravings for high-fat, high-sugar foods to replenish all of that energy we just used.

Problem is, these days we don't have big ol' scary creatures chasing us. Instead, we have bills to pay, relationships to manage, and overflowing inboxes to wrangle. And while all of these responsibilities can feel like a beast at our door, the tasks don't require huge bursts of physical energy to manage. (Although it may *feel* like you're conquering sabertooth tigers now and again.) So although we're not facing *physical* stresses, the way our body reacts hasn't evolved to know the difference between mental and physical stress. And so with a last-minute work deadline or other anxiety-producing event, we get a huge rush of get-it-done-*now* energy (*I haven't eaten in hours and feel fine!*), followed by a period of cravings for less-than-healthy eats (*OMG, I could eat a whole cheesecake and need to sleep for a week*). Obviously, it's much harder to make healthy decisions and stay at a healthy weight when your body is all stressed out.

And what makes this whole fight-or-flight response even worse in these modern, non-cavewoman days is that many of us don't just get stressed a time or two a month—we are *chronically* stressed. This means that our stress hormones are perpetually high. Sorry to be the bearer of bad (and, ironically, potentially stressful) news, but sometimes you have to know the truth before you can really feel compelled to take the time to de-stress. Stress has huge effects

SEVEN STRESS-BUSTING SUPERFOODS

Check out these seven foods that help kick stress to the curb.

1. Avocado. We're pretty much obsessed with the creamy, filling avocado. In addition to having plenty of healthy fats, this little green fruit (yes, it's technically a fruit!) is rich in glutathione, which helps block intestinal absorption of certain fats that cause stress to your system. Enjoy it on sandwiches, in salads, or even sliced with a few pieces of nitrate-free deli turkey. Yum . . .

2. Dark chocolate. Just another reason to love dark chocolate! It's high in flavonoids, which can have a relaxing effect on the body, and phenethylamine, a chemical that has been shown to boost mood. And the darker the better, so go for 70 percent cacao or higher!

3. Oatmeal. Having a morning bowl of oats can be a great way to start the day stress-free. Whole-grain carbs like those found in oatmeal help your body to produce serotonin, which gives your mood a boost (and a happy state of mind always helps challenging situations seem less challenging!) and helps keep your blood sugar levels stable.

4. Berries. Be it blueberries, strawberries, raspberries, or blackberries, all berries rock. Besides having high antioxidant levels, they are rich in vitamin C, which has been shown to help combat stress. Also, they're the perfect topping on your stress-busting oatmeal!

5. Salmon. High in omega-3 fatty acids, salmon boosts serotonin levels and can help suppress the production of adrenaline and cortisol. We like it grilled, poached, steamed, or baked. Or in burgers. Really, just eat it!

6. Nuts. We're nutty for nuts of all kinds! A great mix of protein and fat, nuts are an energizing snack and a good source of zinc, which helps fight anxiety and depression. Because our bodies have no way of storing zinc, it's important to have a small handful of nuts just about every day. Enjoy them in trail mix, in salads, as a crunchy topping to roasted veggies or soup, or on that morning bowl of stress-fighting oatmeal we keep going on and on about.

7. Spinach. Popeye was right to eat his spinach! Leafy greens like spinach are high in magnesium, which helps improve your body's response to stress. Whether it's raw in a salad, sautéed with some garlic, or sneaked into your morning smoothie, load up on spinach!

on every aspect of your well-being, so de-stressing isn't something you "should" make time for—it's something that you *must* make a priority in order to live the longest, healthiest life possible. It's super important and integral to being an FBG!

Why Workouts Beat Stress

Throughout the book you've heard us say that you should leave a workout feeling energized, refreshed, and full of vigor. You know that workouts are great at pumping out those feel-good endorphins. And this is one of the reasons workouts are amazing at beating stress. It's almost like the restart button for your mood. Workouts can help (literally) burn off stress so that you can chill out.

There are about a million types of workouts, and all of them do something to help with stress—namely, because exercise causes your body to release feel-good endorphins into your bloodstream. And feeling good is pretty much the opposite of being stressed. Those steady-state cardio workouts you're doing? They are darn near cathartic and serve as a kind of moving meditation. With each step and movement, you are simply shedding the stress of the day. Those HIIT sessions? They're so intense that you simply can't think about anything but what you're doing in that immediate moment, so you get a nice break from the worries of the day. Heck, even strength training fights stress by making your entire body stronger and more apt to make the physical tasks in your life less taxing. Not to mention that it's hard to fret about the day's events when you're focusing on lifting something heavy with good form.

All of the flexibility workouts—stretching, yoga, Pilates—are particularly good for beating stress, too. Each of them has a relaxed, mindful component to it, which research has shown is good for reducing cortisol levels, improving sleep, and helping you to feel less frazzled. In addition to stretching out the body, these mind-body workouts help to stretch the mind by encouraging exercisers to find internal and external balance, achieve better focus, respect their bodies, and love themselves unconditionally.

No matter what workout you do, make it an opportunity to get away from the worries of your world. When you see workouts as "me time" and something that you enjoy, they're even more likely to help you beat stress. So when you're feeling particularly stressed out—even when you don't think you have the time to work out—get active. In fact, those are the most important days to work out. Listen to your intuition and ask yourself what kind of workout will help you to feel better. Whether it's some yoga, Tai Chi, or intervals on the treadie, do it for you!

ENERGIZE!
Watch Your Caffeine Intake

When your energy is low because you didn't sleep as much as you'd have liked to, it can be tempting to hit the coffeepot, again and again. But while caffeine can give you a temporary jolt of energy, it won't feel so great when it wears off. So while we do enjoy some morning Joe, we recommend limiting it to just one or two cups (which is 8 to 16 ounces—not one of those mega venti cups!)—or, better yet, try green tea or water instead.

The Sleep and Weight Connection

Glorious, glorious sleep. Can we all agree that getting a good night's sleep is awesome for helping us feel refreshed and energized? Thought so. But did you also know that getting enough good-quality sleep can help to keep you at a healthy weight? True story: not sleeping enough has been linked to weight gain and difficulty in losing weight for those who have pounds to lose—namely, because not getting enough sleep is a form of stress.

Sadly, most of us don't get the recommended seven to nine hours of sleep a night for optimum health. In fact, many of us—all stressed out and trying to cram too much into a single day—are what health professionals call "short sleepers," or those who only get five and a half to six hours of shut-eye a night. Half-zombie/half-women, we short-sleepers aren't just walking around tired, we're actually hurting our healthy living goals by skimping on the zzz's.

The connection between sleep and weight is fourfold. First, when we sleep less, we don't burn as many calories. Researchers aren't clear on whether this is due to a drop in metabolism or if it's just because we're so tired that we don't move as much as we do when we're rested; either way, when we don't sleep enough we don't expend as much energy. And that planned trip to the gym? Well, you probably feel too tired to go.

Second, when we sleep less, we eat more. When we don't get enough sleep, we have more frequent and more intense cravings. Not to mention that when you're exhausted, you start eyeballing anything that might give you an energy jolt. That includes the do-nuts in the break room and the caffeine-filled sugary coffee drink; you try to do what it takes to keep yourself going, even if you know it's not good for you. In fact, in one study, women who clocked only four hours of sleep ate several hundred more calories the next day than they did after getting nine hours of sleep. So much so that it added up to about a pound of weight gain in less than two weeks. Yeowsers.

Third, skimping on sleep may cause your body to get stubborn about storing fat. When sleep deprived, your body is more likely to retain fat, even when you're doing all the right things like eating right and working out. This, in layman's terms, means that not sleeping enough makes it harder for you to lose weight.

Last but not least? When you sleep less you have more time to nosh! Yes, you may have more hours to get things done, but you also have more hours to eat. Anyone who's eaten a fourth meal in the day totally knows this one is true. And just think of all those times when you weren't really hungry but ended up mindlessly munching in front of the TV instead of hitting the hay early. Simply put, the more hours you are awake, the more energy your body needs to function.

When you have a lot to do (and who doesn't?!), it may seem like sleep is the one negotiable part of your day that you can short-change. But for all of the reasons above, we urge you not to. Getting good sleep isn't a luxury (although it may certainly feel like it sometimes). It's a necessity! And setting bedtime as a nonnegotiable time sometimes has the mysterious power of cutting down on procrastination as we better organize our time so that we're more efficient. Sure, we may miss a few episodes of reality TV, but that's a small price to pay for being healthier and having more energy!

FIT BOTTOMED MANTRA

"The time to relax is when you don't have time for it."
—SYDNEY J. HARRIS

Putting Things in Perspective

It's so important to calm down and chill out. But we know that not all stress is avoidable. We all have things outside of our control that we have to do and deal with. Stress, problems, and craziness are just a part of life. However, you get to choose how you respond to it—and how you frame your thinking. Harkening back to Chapter 5 on focusing on the positives, it's super important to put any stressful situation in the right perspective.

In many ways, we create our own stress. We put too much pressure on ourselves. We expect ourselves to be perfect. We're afraid to make mistakes, or look stupid, or even be fully ourselves. Rather than living in the present, we're thinking too much about the past or focusing too much on the future. We are not fully conscious in the current moment—and even if we are, we're wishing things were different. Really, the true definition of stress is not accepting things as they are—and wishing something was different.

You've got just one life. So you have to ask yourself: Is it really worth it to spend so much time worrying and stressed out? Are there things you could give up? Do you secretly kind of like rushing around and being stressed out? Or are you wasting your life away by wishing that some magical fairy would come take away all of life's little problems with a little flick of her wand instead of choosing to be happy and calm now? Get honest with yourself. And then use our 10-Minute Fixes to chill out!

Stress fixes

Now that we've convinced you to kick a little stress to the curb, we're going to walk you through exactly how to do it. After all, we don't want to stress you out by making you figure out how to de-stress! Try these 10-minute relaxation breaks for instant Zen that'll pay you back tenfold. Get it? "Ten"-fold.

(1) **PINPOINT NEGATIVE STRESS.** Not *all* stress is bad stress. Stress helps motivate us to get that big work project done and away from threatening situations (like that sabertooth tiger). But too much of the bad stress is *no bueno*. So take 10 minutes to identify the major stressors in your life and devise a plan to make them less stressful.

Step 1: Find it. Go through your typical day in your head. Write down the times you feel stressed. Is it in the rushed mornings? Is it a daily task at work? Is it figuring out what on earth to make for dinner? Make a list of all the places and times in your life where you start kicking into stress mode.

Step 2: Dig deeper. Ask yourself: Why are those times stressful? Pinpoint the reasons big and small as to why exactly those stressors occur. Is it because you don't have enough time? Are you procrastinating? Taking on too much? Could you streamline your day or be more organized?

Step 3: Fix it. Ask yourself the following questions: Which aspects of the stressful situation are in your control? What would make the situation less stressful for you? Are there other people who could help alleviate the stress? Are there things you could do to change how those situations unfold? Once you pinpoint the exact cause of the stress and how it's in your control, you can work to fix it. Make plans before the stress crops up again, so you'll know how to react in the frazzled moment.

Here are a few examples of stressors and how to implement changes for the better!

STRESS 1: WHAT DO I MAKE FOR DINNER?

Dig deeper: Your chronic lack of dinner preparations leave you scrambling for meals and grabbing unhealthy options.

Stress-reducing fix: Set up a plan of attack. Plan a weekly menu and do grocery shopping every Sunday, or have quick 10-minute backup meals ready when you're short on time.

STRESS 2: THE MORNING RUSH

Dig deeper: Styling your fabulous self in the morning never allows for enough time to get out the door on time with a healthy breakfast in your belly.

Stress-reducing fix: Try choosing your outfit the night before so you're not in a rush. Have a quick breakfast ready that you can take on the go, like trail mix or a protein bar and fruit.

STRESS 3: CLUTTER HAS YOU CLIMBING THE WALLS

Dig deeper: No time to clean leaves you with piles of stuff that take over every room.

Stress-reducing fix: Banish all of the bulk, whether it's by having a "clutter box" in each room or by having a designated day of the week when you streamline your belongings.

10-Minute Fixes

(2) SHOWER YOURSELF WITH RELAXATION. When you're in the midst of a stressful week and just need a break, step away and shower yourself with relaxation. Turn your next shower into *om* time by making it your mission to relax and pamper yourself. Play soothing music and light your favorite scented candle. Invest in a luxurious body scrub, a yummy soap, or a hair treatment that will make you feel like you're at a spa. As you shampoo your hair, take an extra minute to really massage your scalp. As you exfoliate your feet, give them a really deep rub. Be mindful of every drop of water that comes out of the showerhead and lands on your body. For a full 10 minutes, imagine the water washing away your troubles and worries, and feel your body relaxing as the warmth soothes any physical tension in your body. Remember to breathe, and you'll be de-stressed (and clean) in no time!

(3) DO A YOGA SERIES. If you're feeling the stress in your shoulders at the end of a long day or just want to do a quick unwind midday, this quick yoga series will give you a good stretch and a bit of relaxing energy. Plus, it'll stretch out those spots where you hold a lot of tension, like your back, shoulders, and hips!

- **Standing forward bend:** Start by standing, knees slightly bent, and swoop your arms down to the ground, bending at your waist to a standing forward bend. Breathe deeply for five breaths. Feel the stretch in your hamstrings as the tension leaves your back and shoulders.
- **Downward-facing dog:** From the forward bend, place your hands firmly on the ground in front of you and step back with your feet

until you're in an inverted V position. This will strengthen your upper body while giving your hamstrings a nice stretch. Breathe deeply here for another five breaths.

- **Cat-cow:** From downward dog, bend your knees and come down onto all fours in a tabletop position. Arch your back and look toward the sky before rounding your back like a cat. Breathe with your movement here and alternate between cat-cow five times. This posture allows you to release the tension you're holding in your chest, shoulders, and back.
- **Child's pose:** From cat-cow, drop your fit bottom back toward your heels and stretch your arms overhead, palms on the ground. Breathe here for five breaths. This is great for the back and shoulders and for stretching the hips.

Repeat this segment a couple of times. If you have a spare minute, lie down in corpse pose to end with a few deep breaths. Then feel the calm energy!

(4) **COOK A HEALTHY MEAL MINDFULLY.** Next time you start to make dinner, don't view it as yet another task on your list. Instead, try to enjoy the process. If you're the type of person who hates cooking, make it a point to stop the negative mental chatter and focus on the positives of the experience. Find a healthy recipe you're excited about making. Put on some fun tunes, pour yourself a glass of wine or some sparkling water, and use your fancy stemware—it might just be Tuesday, but make it feel like an occasion!

Pay attention to all of your senses as you make your culinary creation, and don't be afraid to pretend you're on a cooking show. Look at the beautiful produce; carefully measure the grains of rice or quinoa. Pay attention to the feel of a tomato in your hand. Feel the spray of citrus as you peel an orange. Smell the fresh herbs as you chop them. Listen to the snap of snow peas and the sizzle of peppers as you drop them into a skillet to sauté. Taste the ingredients as you put your healthy meal together. Let the process of cooking become a sensory experience, enjoying every sight and sound, even the rhythm of chopping.

Work on being totally present—focus on the task at hand and forget about what's on your to-do list. (Plus, sharp knives and distractions don't go well together anyway.) When you sit down to eat, think about how the nutrients will give you the fuel you need for your workouts and your life. Then eat your meal as mindfully as you made it.

5 **TRY A SELF-MASSAGE.** Grab a clean tennis ball and roll the arches of your bare feet on it for an instant feel-good boost. After a couple of minutes of that, do the same with the palms of your hands. Next, take your fingertips and gently massage your temples, forehead, cheeks, and earlobes in a tight, circular motion. Then, with a larger circular motion, give yourself a head massage. If you have time, grab a massage oil or lotion and massage your hands and feet, paying particular attention to your fingers and toes. Rub your shoulders, arms, and legs if you have time to spare. While a dedicated hour with a massage therapist is always amazing, you'll be surprised at how good self-massage can feel!

6 **PROGRESSIVELY RELAX.** It might seem counterintuitive to tense your muscles to relax, but give this progressive relaxation

exercise a try. By purposefully tensing your muscles and consciously releasing them, you'll help yourself relax and release
tension that was living there.

Find a quiet place and either lie down or sit comfortably.
Working from toe to head, tense your muscles for a few seconds
and then relax them and feel tension melt away. Tense your
feet, then move up to your calves, knees, and thighs. Tense your
butt muscles, your back. Tense and release your fingers, arms,
then shoulders. Tense your neck, jaw, cheeks, and forehead. Go
slowly, tensing and releasing all of the muscles of your body. As
you release the tension from each muscle, imagine your stress
melting away with the release, taking deep breaths the whole
time. Ahhh . . .

(7) **GET A BETTER NIGHT'S SLEEP.** Whether you think you're sleeping like a baby at night or you think your sleep could use some
improvement, take 10 minutes to check out your sleep environment and make sure you're promoting the best night's sleep you
can get.

Check the nightstand: Is your cell phone there? iPad? Laptop?
Playing on your electronic devices and hearing dings from new
texts or emails can distract you from hitting the hay when you
should. Even low-tech options like books can prove distracting
and keep you up late. Experts recommend using your bed only
for sleeping and doing the horizontal hokey-pokey, so read
that last chapter on the couch, leave your phone in another
room, and turn off the computer before you get in bed. Make
sure your sleep environment is sufficiently dark, too, as light

will wake you up and make you feel alert. (Which is another reason you should keep the phone away from bed and consider covering the bright light of your alarm clock!)

Listen up: Take a moment to listen to your sleep environment. Is there a ticking clock? A dripping faucet? A roommate or partner watching TV until all hours of the night? Limit the noises you can, and then for those sounds that are outside of your control, buy a fan or a white noise machine that will drown out distracting sounds and lull you to dreamland. There are even apps for that—just make sure you're following the "no distractions" rule.

Implement a pre-sleep ritual: The right nighttime ritual will help you relax and wind down for a restful night's sleep. Start with a cup of soothing chamomile tea in the hour before bedtime. Once you're done sipping, lather yourself with a lavender-scented lotion, and then spritz your bed linens with a mist of lavender spray. (Both lavender and chamomile are said to aid sleep.) Finish up your bedtime routine with 10 deep breaths while seated on your bed to ease into bedtime.

Rituals like these are a fun way to create a healthy habit. Do them often and you'll even start to associate your tea and lavender with the winding-down process, so as soon as you taste or smell them, you'll start chillaxing.

(8) **GET MINDFUL AND MEDITATE.** While you can read endless books on the art of meditation and attend classes, there is no need for anything complicated, which is why we've put together this super-simple 10-minute meditation. Don't get hung up on the "right" way to meditate—there is no right or wrong here. You

can do this meditation at any time of the day. If you regularly get stressed at work and turn to munching, a time-out for deep breathing can help curb that habit. You can also do it in the morning to gear up for the day, or it can be the last thing you do before you hit the hay at night (although your meditation may run short if you fall asleep).

Set an alarm for 10 minutes (unless it's bedtime) and get comfortable. That can be sitting on the floor or in bed with your legs crossed or lying down; you make the rules. Then spend the next 10 minutes breathing. Clear your thoughts as much as you can and focus on breathing deeply and exhaling fully. Each time a thought appears, let it slip away with your breath. Focus on releasing tension with the breath. You can even repeat an affirmation like "calm" or "relax" as you breathe to help you focus your intentions. Moving from your feet to your head, breathe into each part of your body, releasing tension with each breath as you go. When your alarm goes off, take one last breath and open your eyes to greet the day again, carrying your sense of Zen with you wherever you go!

9 **REMEMBER TO BREATHE.** Breathing. You do it all day, every day, but much like swallowing or blinking, you don't really think about this necessary bodily function. When you take the time to pay attention to breathing, however, you can feel noticeable stress release and calm. Studies have even shown that correct breathing can help with chronic conditions like hypertension, asthma, and panic attacks and even lower blood pressure and reduce stress. Some studies show that it can slow down the heart rate, relax muscles, and calm the mind.

Take 10 minutes to set breathing reminders throughout your day. It can be a reoccurring alarm on your cell phone, a pop-up appointment on your computer, or a sticky note on the bathroom mirror reminding you to stop and breathe. It can even be a mental note that every hour on the hour, you take a moment to focus on your breath. When you see those reminders, stop what you're doing and take a few deep breaths.

This is also a good time to pay attention to your posture and to make sure you're breathing correctly. Sit up straight with your shoulders relaxed and down. When you're just starting out, place a hand on the belly and allow the deep breath to let your abdomen expand. You should feel the belly rise. Then exhale fully, feeling your tension melt away. Aim to inhale for three counts, hold for three counts, and then exhale for three counts.

(10) JOURNAL YOUR RESPONSE: *Why I deserve to take care of myself.* If we haven't convinced you to slow down and de-stress, you're going to convince yourself with this journal exercise. For the next 10 minutes, explore why you deserve to take care of yourself. How do you deserve to be treated by yourself? Why are you worthy of pampering? How do you feel when you're relaxed and properly taking care of yourself? Who does it allow you to be?

It's probably not often that you actually think about how you take care of yourself—how you take time to unwind and how important that is for you to feel your best. So after you write, take a few minutes to read back over your writing. Try to keep the insights you wrote down top-of-mind so that you're motivated to take time to chill out.

CHAPTER 8

Help a Sister Out

By now you know how awesome it is to incorporate all of these healthy tweaks into your life. And as awesome and empowering as that is, there is something that can take it to the next level: helping others do the same! We love sharing our favorite healthy tips and tricks with others—obviously, or we wouldn't have started a website or be writing this book to do so. Whether it's a tasty recipe, getting a team together to raise money for a good cause, being supportive of a workout buddy, or sharing our latest goof at the gym, helping others and spreading the FBG love is so inspiring and motivating.

Building a supportive, active network—whether it's one person strong or ten deep—gives you workout buddies, people to share tricks with, and buds who can inspire you. Not only that, but others will hold you accountable to your goals and keep you motivated to push yourself even when you'd rather take it easy. It's also more fun to do things with friends; they can give you the confidence to try things you might be too intimidated to try by yourself—there is safety in numbers, after all. So that trapeze course, dance class, or even that date to go walk at the track? Your friend will make sure you show up—and have a blast while you're doing it.

We've got tons of ideas for you on how to expand your network of fit friends and cultivate supportive relationships. Likewise, we'll help you deal with those who might not jump on the healthy living bandwagon—and even those who sabotage your efforts. Our 10-Minute Fixes are all about helping others, spreading the FBG love, and helping a sister out. Because when you help others, you help yourself!

Strong Support

Friendships make life more awesome. And, as you've probably noticed, we're all about the awesome. But there is a difference between a healthy friendship and a not-so-healthy friendship. By no means does a friend have to be a carbon copy of you (hey, differences make the world go round!), but it does help to have friends who have similar goals and pursuits—especially when it comes to a healthy lifestyle. But, as you're growing and changing, it can sometimes be difficult to find others who share your ambitions to change. Then what? Do you try to include those people in your life on your journey, or do you try to find new fit friends? We recommend doing a little bit of both.

It goes without saying that all friends should be supportive, encouraging, honest—and want the best for you. If you have unhealthy or unfit friends who fit this bill, it's worth trying to include them on this journey. While they may not be as ready to change as you are, it certainly doesn't hurt to invite them on some of the beginner-friendly healthy pursuits you're doing. Things like checking out the farmer's market, going for a walk around the park, or cooking healthy meals together are all good options. Just as we've taught you to embrace the positives of living a healthy life for good, try to emphasize the same principles to them. Make it as fun and normal as you can, and be patient if they're not super receptive. Remember, we're all on our own journeys here, and everyone is a little different. Respect their decisions, but be honest about why this journey is important to you; make it clear that you'd like to include them, but that you're committed to making a change either way. Even if they aren't ready to join your efforts 100 percent, tell them how best to support you; after all, real friendships are about honesty, give-and-take, and a whole lot of love!

The Saboteurs

Just because you've taken the FBG healthy track doesn't mean that everyone in your life will be eating kale and doing push-ups during prime-time TV viewing. Sure, your loved ones are likely to think it's great that you're getting healthier. But they may also worry about the impact your new habits will have on them. Your hubby may worry he's going to be eating lettuce for dinner every night. Your BFF might worry that she'll lose you to your new yoga buddies. Your mom might mourn your weekly coffee and pastry date. Your work buds might be sad you're skipping happy hours for an hour at the gym. Sometimes, saboteurs are simply defensive about their own less-than-healthy habits—and sometimes are not even fully aware that they're trying to drag you down.

Saboteurs can take all forms. Sometimes people can unintentionally sabotage you when they actually think they're being supportive—think of those who urge you to splurge on a dessert because you "deserve it!" But things can get tricky if you do have a friend who refuses to support you, or as we mentioned previously, begins to sabotage you or bring you down. Any friend who makes you feel bad about yourself or doesn't want the best for you is not a real friend. And while it may be hard to do, breaking up with a toxic friend—or drastically cutting how much time you see the person—may be a necessity. Just as you're learning to put nutritious foods in your body and move your body so that it feels its best, you have to cultivate and maintain relationships that are just as good for your soul.

Best Fit Friends

Before you embark on a new healthy lifestyle, have a conversation with the people most important to you—romantic partners and close family members are typically the best support systems (and most likely offenders!). Simply ask for their support up front and bring up any issues or joint habits you've fallen into that may get in the way of your goals. Share with them the goals you have, and come up with concrete ways for them to support you, whether it's to go for a walk with you or be a guinea pig for your new healthy recipes. It can be tough to rock the boat and to go against old, established habits, but it's worth creating some waves when it comes to improving your health. Those who truly love you will want what's best and healthiest for you.

A little bit of shifting in relationships is probably inevitable, too, particularly if you've created unhealthy habits with close friends and family members; we all have the friends we bond with over bottles of wine or indulgent dinners out. If you have friends who are really unsupportive, don't feel bad about spending less time with them and setting boundaries. Studies have actually shown that obesity is, in a way, contagious. In fact, one study found that when a friend became obese, your odds of becoming obese increase by 57 percent. Encouragingly, though, the same effect actually occurred for weight loss, too, so it is possible to inspire those around you with your healthy habits.

Healthy living sabotage can manifest in a lot of different ways. It can be as simple as a friend offering—insistently—that you try her Super-Duper Double Fudge Brownie Sundae Cake. It can be that your husband teases you when he sees you rocking out to a workout DVD. Maybe your best friend pouts because you stopped splitting dessert after dinners out. But no matter what form it takes, know that it's not really about you, so don't take it personally.

Knowing some of the reasons people can sabotage you can help you combat it and increase your odds of sticking with the anti-diet way of life you love. Reminding yourself of your goals—and accomplishments—and the polite but firm "no, thank you" are two of the best tools you have against saboteurs. Own your commitment to yourself. Show them how happy you are and how much better you feel than before. Seeing is believing, and it's hard to argue with an energy-filled Fit Bottomed Girl. Be confident in your choices and don't be afraid to be a little bit stubborn if you have to be. You're totally worth sticking up for!

It's not the number of friends you have that matters, either. While having a large support system can be helpful, if you have a smaller one or even just a friend or two—that's totally okay. When it comes to friendship, it's the quality, not the quantity, that matters. We'd rather you have a really amazing best friend who's always there for you rather than fifty acquaintances who are too busy to chat after a hard day. And don't worry—if you don't have any friends who fit this bill, we have lots and lots of suggestions on how to make new healthy buds a little later!

Leading the Way

In starting to follow the FBG way of life, you actually become a leader. When you're making healthy decisions and feeling generally awesome, it's quite a confidence booster. You'll feel more empowered and in control than ever.

Enthusiasm is contagious, and when you're enthusiastic about your lifestyle and genuinely enjoying all of the healthy and wonderful things you've discovered, people will notice. Others start looking to you for guidance and support. Leading by example and becoming a role model—for a friend, a spouse, your kids, or your parents—happens naturally when you feel good about who you are and how you're living. When you "infect" others with the healthy-living enthusiasm, your support network grows, which is a powerful motivator in itself. When you know others are behind you, rooting for you, it's easier to stay on track. A support network gives you someone to go to if the going gets tough; it gives you someone to cheer for and to cheer for you. It's a circle of inspiration. You inspire others; they inspire you.

Don't feel pressure to be perfect in leading this healthy life. You don't have to be perfect to be a role model or to help others! You can help others out simply by being a good influence. You can show people that having fun and making healthy choices aren't mutually exclusive. Being confident in your decisions and making healthy choices because you want to make healthy choices will go a long

HEALTHY, HAPPY HELPERS

Enlisting friends to accompany you on your Fit Bottomed journey isn't just a feel-good thing to do, although it certainly does feel good. You'll get tangible health benefits when you help others. Really!

Studies have shown that helping others—like volunteering or even doing housework or errands and other tasks for a friend—seems to provide a buffer that protects you from the negative effects of stress. In fact, those who offered support to others experienced dramatic improvements in their quality of life, were significantly happier, and were less depressed than those who didn't. And you don't have to be Mother Teresa and dedicate all of your free time to helping others to reap rewards (remember balance from earlier? Still important!). In one study, just an hour a week was all it took to improve mental and physical health. So help others, and help yourself!

way toward convincing others that this anti-diet way of life is the way to go.

Besides just setting a good example for those closest to you, there are so many other ways to get out there to further inspire others if and when you're feeling that you want to take leadership to the next level. You can start a healthy living group at work, or get together family or co-workers for a weight-loss challenge. Or get involved and lead others in their fitness endeavors with organizations, like Girls on the Run and Fit Girls, which aim to get girls running and moving and build self-esteem and confidence. See if coaches are needed in your area or start a fitness endeavor all your own! Check out our 10-Minute Fixes on more ways to give back, too. The possibilities are endless.

FROM THE FBGs
Thoughts on Giving Back

FROM ERIN: When you read something hilarious, you want to read it out loud to a friend. When you see a funny video on YouTube, you immediately send it to a friend who would appreciate it. When you watch TV, you laugh harder when you're laughing with a loved one. So when you find something that makes you feel healthier and better about your body, you should share that, too! When I find something healthy I love, I want to share it. Maybe people don't know how awesome this exercise class is! Maybe others are intimidated by the assisted pull-up machine, too! Maybe others have never tried Brussels sprouts and need a push to try them!

I give mad props to Jenn for sharing her love of fitness with me. I'd always been active, but her passion for healthy living inspired me and keeps me motivated. She pushed to start FBG, and I got excited to jump on board and give back. She introduced me to Zumba, and now I encourage everyone to try it. (Always. I'm probably annoying about it.) I just feel that someone was kind enough to drag me along to a Zumba class, and it's my duty to share the love and pass it along. It's the circle of fitness fun!

It can be hard to branch out and try new things. But nothing feels quite as good as discovering something new! As a self-appointed FBG ambassador, I feel that I'm doing my job if I help even one person take things not so seriously because I can laugh at myself goofing up or sing the praises of a new recipe loudly enough that they want to try it. Maybe someone will run a 10K because I, someone who is decidedly not a runner, did it, too. Maybe someone will try kale because I shared a delicious way to eat it. If I can inspire someone to flip her thinking to a healthier mentality, to embrace and love herself even more, then I feel even more inspired to keep doing those things in my own life.

Support fixes

Ready to get social and inspire others on your journey to living like an FBG? Check out our 10-Minute Fixes for finding your exercise soul mate (or really good workout buddy), doing your part to make the world a healthier place, and more!

1. **TRANSFORM A BUDDY INTO AN FBG.** You don't have to make a go of your health goals alone. Having a workout buddy can help you work harder and longer, so it is great for your health to partner up (provided you don't push it too hard!). Your contact list has plenty of awesome people already on it, so start putting a health-and-fitness spin on your existing friendships. Take 10 minutes to look at the people in your life and see who would be a great buddy to have along for marathon training, who would be willing to go for a weekly walk in the park, who would be a willing road warrior for biking adventures. Maybe a co-worker has always wanted to try a group exercise class, or maybe a friend who loves to cook would be willing to do a weekly veggie recipe swap. Find a group of friends who would like to have a healthy recipe potluck party. Everyone cooks up a delicious dish, and then you take portions to go so that you have meals ready for the rest of the week! Take 10 minutes to reach out to the people in your life and make some fit plans together.

2. **JOIN THE (HEALTHY) CLUB.** If you need a little extra support from an active community of like-minded fitties, your best bet is to expand your social circle. There are plenty of places to meet and greet those with similar fitness interests, you just have to be willing!

Join a gym: Hit up the local gym for people who are trying to get fit. Group exercise classes are a great way to get to know people; there is reassurance in chatting with people who thought a class was killer, too. Gym bulletin boards are a great place to look for activities, such as group runs or special events or classes.

Spend group time: Join a running club or a cycling group if that's where your interest lies. These types of groups are great if you're a newbie; most enthusiasts love giving tips on their sport!

Rec yourself: Check out your local YMCA or community recreation center for classes, intramural sports, and opportunities to expand your fitness horizons and social circle.

Take a cooking class: Learn to whip up a healthy meal while you mingle with peeps who are doing the same. If you find a few you'd like to know better, organize a healthy potluck party!

Start a get-fit challenge: Don't think you have to follow and join in others' groups—start one yourself! Whether it's a group to train for a race, or a competition to lose a few inches, poll your co-workers and extended fam to see who would be up for the challenge!

Head online: Whether it's a community like SparkPeople or a forum dedicated to your fitness forte, there are gobs and gobs of online options for friendship. So whether you prefer to make online friends for daily support or prefer to go to Meetup.com, where you can turn common interests into real-life friendships, peek around the interwebs to find a quality fit friend—or an entire community of them.

(3) **CREATE A HEALTHY ONLINE RECIPE COLLECTION.** Because eating awesome, healthy yumminess is so key to the FBG lifestyle, it's important to stay inspired in the kitchen. Which means seeking out delicious new recipes. Take 10 minutes to start an online recipe collection you can share with friends. Want an easy way to collect ideas and share them at once? Pinterest! Not only are there a zillion recipes and food ideas, but you can connect with friends online and get their ideas, too. Search "healthy recipes" or "easy veggies" for tons of good ideas. Or decide on a specific ingredient you'd like to use and plug it in; it's an easy way to find tons of ways to incorporate a new-to-you ingredient!

Want more healthy-cooking places to look? Major magazines like *EatingWell* and *Cooking Light* have fabulous ideas that can help you keep it fresh in the kitchen. And blogs—don't even get us started on the many, many inspiring healthy-cooking blogs out there. (FitBottomedEats.com comes to mind!) Once you find recipes, don't just let them sit online—use them! Aim to try a new dish every couple of weeks so you can find awesome eats to add to your recipe book. You can even set up a healthy meal exchange: you cook a meal and invite a friend over, and vice versa. Double the recipe tasting with half the work!

(4) **FIND AN ACTIVE VOLUNTEER OPPORTUNITY.** When you sign up to volunteer, you help others. When you sign up for an active volunteering endeavor, you help others while you get some exercise. It's a win-win! Head to serve.gov to search volunteer opportunities in your area. Once you land on something you think you'd like to do, contact the organization to see how you can pitch in. Then actually set a date and get there. Use these

10 minutes to take those first steps to get going! Here are a few active volunteering ideas we love to get you started.

Habitat for Humanity: Ever built a house? A guaranteed workout.

Cleanup: Highway, beach, and park cleanup programs will have you walking while getting some fresh air and helping Mother Nature keep her house clean. Look into national parks for opportunities building trails and other volunteering options.

Anything with kids: Whether it's youth recreation services or Girl Scouts, no matter what you do with kids, they are bound to wear you out!

Soup kitchen: Whether you're cooking up a storm, chopping veggies, or serving those in need, you'll keep moving at a soup kitchen.

Food bank: Sorting and packing food and helping with community food drives will have you helping others while keeping you moving.

Helping at a charity walk/run: If you don't feel comfortable participating in a racing event, volunteer instead. Not only will you be helping the runners and teams get through the race, but you'll be inspired to work your bod, too!

(5) CRASH A FRIEND'S WORKOUT. Party and wedding crashers may not be welcome guests, but workout crashers? Well, we kind of love those. After all, when it comes to getting active, we say the more the merrier! So for this 10-Minute Fix we're going to walk you through crashing a friend's workout.

First, identify the people in your life who do active pursuits that you're interested in trying. It can be anything from joining their running group to trying a new workout class or going hiking or doing a sport—anything! And remember, if it's an activity that scares you a little bit, that's okay! Being a little afraid and facing that fear is a good way to bust out of your comfort zone and find new things you love.

Once you have your list of people, take a couple minutes to give them a call or email them and ask when they're doing said activity next. Explain that you're focusing on getting healthier and trying new things and would love if they could share their experience with you. Might you join them? When you do, what do you need to know and what should you bring? Set a time and crash that workout!

And a fun thing to do after the workout? Send them a nice follow-up thank-you and invite them to join you for one of your favorite workouts.

6 **SEND YOUR WORKOUT BUDDY SOME LOVE!** One of the best ways to motivate yourself is to motivate others. So in order to keep yourself inspired, set aside 10 minutes to send your workout buddy or fellow FBG some extra encouragement.

Tell the person how you're proud of her progress. Shoot the friend an inspirational image or quote you saw online that made you think of her. Talk about how much she's motivated you to go after your dreams or goals. Heck, even a simple "You're doing awesome. Keep it up!" can go a long way in making someone else's day, whether it's in an email, a handwritten note, a social media update, or even a text. So set aside 10 minutes to give someone else a boost. And don't be surprised if she does the same for you down the line!

(7) DONATE OR RECYCLE YOUR OLD WORKOUT SHOES. When the tread starts to wear on your sneakers, it's time to invest in new ones. But what's a gal to do with the old ones? Throwing them away just seems so wasteful. Help Mother Nature and others by recycling or donating your kicks to those in need instead of pitching them in the wastebasket!

Donate 'em: If your shoes are gently worn (like, they just didn't fit right or you ended up not being a huge fan of them), give them to a friend with the same shoe size or donate them to a local thrift store. Or consider getting a bunch of extra pairs together from others and send them in to Soles4Souls, which will get them to people who need them due to poverty, natural disasters, and other circumstances. The organization One World Running also gets running shoes onto the feet of people who need them in the United States and around the world. Check it out!

Recycle 'em: If your shoes are past the point of someone else being able to use them (either the supportive cushioning or tread is out, or they're just plain too dirty to feel good about donating), consider giving them to a good cause like Nike's Reuse-a-Shoe. This program accepts shoes of all brands and transforms them into materials that are used to make tracks, indoor basketball courts, fields, and playgrounds. You can drop off your old sneaks at any Nike store or other drop-off location listed on its website.

Whether you want to donate or recycle, take 10 minutes to do some research online or by calling a local running store (they usually know of a good local option) about what makes the most sense for you and your shoes, and then set a plan to do it!

(8) WRITE A THANK-YOU LETTER TO SOMEONE WHO HAS HELPED YOU. Is there someone in your life who has really been there for you—or really helped you to live a healthier life? Take 10 minutes to thank the person by following this simple formula to thank-you-writing perfection—and get you in a really good headspace by reflecting on a time in your life when someone was there for you.

First, think of a person who has made a healthy difference in your life. It can be anyone—a co-worker, your partner, your best friend, your mom, the really nice front desk person at the gym who always greets you with a smile.

Second, think of a specific instance where that person really made a difference in your day or your attitude. How did it make you feel? What did it change? What would you like to tell her about that moment that maybe she's not aware of?

Lastly, get to writing your thank-you note! It doesn't have to be long or detailed, but cover these aspects in this order:

- Thanks for what she has done
- Expression of what it meant to you and your healthy journey
- Relate it to the future in some way, like "I look forward to seeing you at the gym!"
- End it with a friendly "thanks again!" or other signature line, signature, and send off!

Thanking someone feels good, doesn't it? Feel free to do this 10-Minute Fix as often as you wish as a great way to feel good—and do good!

9) MASTER THE ART OF GIVING—AND RECEIVING—COMPLIMENTS. Do you give compliments often? Do you really *mean* them? What do you usually say when someone gives you a compliment? Do you downplay it or try to counteract it? There is a subtle art to giving and receiving compliments, and unfortunately, most of us aren't *super* good at it. Here's a quick way to start giving genuine compliments, as well as how to accept them with grace so that they always feel good!

Giving compliments: Honesty goes a long way. And people usually know when you're being genuine and when you're not. So the no. 1 step to giving a good compliment is to be sincere. Next, get specific about what you like. If you like someone's hair, is it the color? The cut? The shine? Tell someone what you really, really like about it. If it makes sense, also include what effect it has. And to keep the conversation going and natural, tack on a question—something like "Wow, the color of your hair looks fantastic. It's really beautiful in the sunlight. Where do you get your hair done?" That sure is a lot more interesting, sincere, and conversation-provoking than "I like your hair."

And a couple of quick do-not-dos for giving compliments? Avoid comparisons and don't expect anything in return. Keep it focused on the person and don't make it about anyone else, including yourself. Do these things and you'll definitely help to make someone's day, which is always a feel-good!

Accepting compliments: What is it about compliments that make us feel so darn uncomfortable? Or that make us want to immediately discredit them? Argh! We see women do this time and time again, so let's put an end to the compliment insanity. Believe us: you are worthy of compliments, and by accepting a compliment graciously you will not come off as cocky or arrogant. You will come off as the beautiful, self-assured, and appreciative person you are.

The no. 1 one way to do this is to stop doing any of the following: putting yourself down, thinking that the other person doesn't really mean it, deflecting the compliment to someone else, or disregarding it and bringing up your weaknesses. Right now, take a second and commit to stopping the practice of all of these things. Because, besides bringing yourself down, they're also not very respectful of the very nice thing someone else is saying to you, right?

Then own your accomplishments! You are worthy of praise, be it for your actions, or your attitude, or your outfit, or your hair. You are gorgeous and someone is noticing, and that's awesome! So be appreciative; say a simple thank-you and even a quick bit on what that means to you or how that makes you feel. (And we hope, if the person knows how to give a really great compliment, you'll have a question to answer, too!) It doesn't have to be long-winded or detailed, but feel confident about accepting the compliment.

It may take some practice and time, but giving and receiving compliments is a great way to practice owning your awesomeness and helping others to see how amazing they are, too. Embrace and spread the positivity!

(10) JOURNAL YOUR RESPONSE: *How I am a role model for others.* By now you're on board with how helping others out actually helps us all out, too. But for this journal assignment, we want you to dig deeper into how this applies to *your* life. And we want you to start seeing all of the different ways in which others may look to you for guidance. So set that timer for 10 minutes, take a couple of deep breaths to clear your mind, and begin writing about how you are a role model for others. Who might look up to you? Who asks you for advice? Do you have kiddos in your life who might try to emulate your actions now or in the future? Any co-workers who take an interest in what you're eating, drinking, or doing? How does this make you feel? Do you wish there were others who looked up to you? How could you consciously be a healthier role model?

No matter where you are in your fit journey, know that— even if you're not aware of it—there are others who are watching what you're doing and your healthy habits may be rubbing off on them, even if it takes some time. No FBG is an island!

CHAPTER 9

Laugh at Yourself

Laughter. It truly is the best medicine, right? There is nothing quite like giggling with girlfriends or watching that online video that makes you laugh until your stomach hurts every time. After a rough day, a good laugh can melt your stresses away and erase tension, even if just for a moment. That's why in this chapter, we insist on kicking the serious to the curb. We want you not only to laugh more but also to translate that mentality into how you're treating yourself and how you approach life.

We want you to embrace your inner goofball and to cut yourself some slack—and allow yourself to really be *you,* no matter how silly you look. Because if you haven't discovered it for yourself by now, we'll tell you: you rock. And we think the ability to laugh—especially at yourself—is the key to accepting yourself and really celebrating your uniqueness.

If you're letting a too-serious attitude keep you from having a total blast, we're going to remedy that situation. We want you to stop looking for approval from others and start looking for approval from yourself. We're going to help you unearth your uniquely awesome qualities that make you *you* and help you to find joy in everything you do.

Consider us your giggle guides in this chapter, as we help you implement strategies to up your happiness quotient, to laugh more, and to embrace the silly side of life. We guarantee you'll feel happier and more energized after this chapter! It'll get you laughing, help you embrace your inner goofball, and help you enjoy workouts—and life—just a bit more.

The Importance of Laughter

Laughter just feels good from head to toe—but why? What makes it actually feel good and trigger those happy emotions? Research shows that the muscles you use to laugh actually trigger endorphins, those brain chemicals known for their mood-boosting effects. Research has shown that laughter reduces stress, boosts immunity, and improves blood flow to the heart. A good laugh can even make you feel less pain and sleep better. Smiling has positive benefits on your mood and stress levels, too.

Are people less likely to get sick because they laugh, or do healthy people simply have more reasons to chuckle? Researchers aren't sure. And some experts believe that because laughter is often social, the benefits are really from the social connection and from being around friends (hey, even more reason to pay attention to Chapter 8!). But regardless of the science, laughing certainly makes life more enjoyable. Life is too short to be too serious, especially when happiness feels so good. It's one of the reasons we insist on

LAUGHING IS THE NEW AB WORKOUT

Here's one heck of a reason to get laughing: it actually works your abs. You've probably felt this effect from a really good hysterical-laughing session with your friends, but when you really get to laughing—like the kind where you can't talk or the water you're drinking inadvertently and embarrassingly squirts out of your nose—your ab muscles work hard.

When you laugh, the muscles in your stomach expand and contract, which is basically the same thing they do when you do other ab moves like crunches and sit-ups. And, if you really get to cracking up for more than just a couple of minutes, your heart rate can even get high enough to give you the same benefits as a cardio session. In fact, a full-bellied laugh is comparable to walking at a slow to moderate pace.

adding the fun into fitness; it's one of the reasons our website has a silly name. It's one of the reasons that one of the principles of being a Fit Bottomed Girl is to laugh—and laugh at yourself.

The Seven Keys to Happiness

What really makes us happy? We all want more laughter and joy in our lives. In fact, if you ask most people how they want to feel, the answer is probably "happy" or some form of that. And that makes sense. When we feel happy—whether it's when we're cracking up with a friend, or dancing to our favorite tunes, or just cruising around town with the wind in our hair—we feel good. And we all like to feel good. But what is it that *really* makes us happy? Is it money? Having free time? Seeing the world through rose-colored glasses?

1. **HAVE THE BASICS COVERED.** While, in general, having more stuff won't make you happy, it's common sense that you have to have your basic needs met in order to experience happiness. So you need shelter, food, and clothes on your back. But will twenty pairs of stilettos boost your happiness? Probably not for more than a day or two. Especially once you get the credit card bill!

2. **GET SOCIAL.** We are truly social creatures, and we are naturally happier when we're around people and in committed relationships. As we say in Chapter 8, no FBG is an island, and when it comes to being happy, it certainly helps to have healthy relationships and an active social life. With friends and loved ones we feel safe, cared for, understood, and—you guessed it—more joyful!

3. **APPRECIATE WHAT YOU HAVE.** We've already gone over the power of being more grateful for what you have, but studies have shown that when you actually want what you have, you're happier. So don't spend your time putting off being happy until you have this or do that; love the life you're living now and delight in making it even better.

4. **FEEL GOOD IN YOUR OWN SKIN.** Scientists have found that more attractive people do tend to be happier. But even if you're not Heidi Klum material (and, ahem, who is except Heidi?!), know that you don't have to be a supermodel to benefit. Just believing that you look great is enough to get you smiling.

5. **EMBRACE YOUR PURPOSE.** Whether it's through religion, spirituality, or just knowing that you are here on this earth for a reason,

embracing your purpose in life can make you feel more fulfilled and—you guessed it—happier.

6. **ENJOY GETTING OLDER.** Many of us dread getting older, but tacking on the years does, according to research, seem to pump up the happiness. As each birthday passes, we really do learn to stop sweating the small stuff and focus on the truly important things in life. Having that perspective, wisdom, and knowledge from years past shows us what really matters. And focusing on that makes us really feel good.

7. **LIVE A HEALTHY LIFESTYLE.** You knew this one was coming, right? We've written a whole book on why this is true (thank you for reading it!), but being active and healthy is shown to increase happiness levels. When you're feeling good, life feels good!

Remember, being happy isn't about being perfect; it's about creating a life that you love and enjoying it to the fullest. No matter where you are in life, you are the one who is in control of her own happiness. And the first step to being happy is to decide that you want to be happy and then center your life on doing the things that bring you joy and make you feel truly good. Being happy is a conscious decision that you get to make every day!

FIT BOTTOMED MANTRA

"A person without a sense of humor is like a wagon without springs. It's jolted by every pebble on the road."

—HENRY WARD BEECHER

Knock It Off with the Serious

It's great to have serious ambition and goals, especially when it comes to fitness. But those goals are going to be painful to meet unless you're having *fun*. Oftentimes, we hold back from trying something new because we're afraid of looking like a fool. Of goofing up. Of looking incompetent. But don't hold back because you're afraid to look silly or make a goofball out of yourself; embrace the inner goofball! Spicing up your fitness routine with different activities is good for your bod because it can also help you find new activities that will aid you in achieving your goals faster. That's along with keeping you more focused because you're enjoying yourself, which means that the time will really fly!

Especially when it comes to exercise, one of the things that can hold people back is being afraid of what others think of them. Whether you're afraid to join a gym because you think everyone there is in better shape or whether you're afraid to take a class because you don't think you'll be able to keep up, we've got news for you: *no one cares*. At least, no one cares nearly as much as you think they do. Think about the last time you were at the grocery store. Did you notice that other person in produce? If you did, how much time did you spend judging what was in her cart? Probably not at all; you had your own shopping to take care of. So how likely is it that there is going to be someone scrutinizing every move you make? They're all probably too focused on what they're doing to pay much attention to anybody else! And, honestly, even if they are getting all judgey in their heads about you, who cares? We are absolutely positive your health and fitness goals are more important than what some hypothetically judgmental gym rat thinks of how you look in your workout clothes or how much weight you're lifting.

FROM THE FBGS
Funniest Fitness Moment

FROM JENN: On our websites, Erin and I have pretty much written about it all: chafing, periods, underwear, sex, pooping—you name it, we've probably covered it. Nothing is really off-limits. So when we got the chance to try a product that allowed women to pee standing up, I knew we had to try it. After all, as someone who loves to camp and backpack, I've long "admired" men's peeing abilities. (You might say I have "pee envy." Men clearly have an advantage when it comes to urinating. It's really not fair.)

Erin and I both received this gizmo, which ended up being kind of like a funnel (in the color pink!) for your lady parts. I tested mine on a summer camping trip, while Erin went a bit more domestic with her review, trying it in the bathroom. These facts in and of themselves were enough humorous material for a post. But once the "going" got going (pun intended), it only got better.

During my camping trip, just a few hours after stepping on a thorn and injuring my foot (which only adds to the ridiculousness of the situation), I hobbled in to try the peeing product. And, despite my throbbing foot, I was excited at the prospect of standing up to go no. 1. So I unzipped my pants, put it on, pushed my hips out, and peed. *Standing up.* Sweet peeing gender-equality, victory was mine. While it felt a bit weird, it was freeing. No more hovering behind a bush, hoping no person or creature walked by! Hooray!

And then I quickly learned that it's easy for the funnel to back up. And back up it did—all over my camping pants. Victory denied. Gross as it was, I could not stop laughing. Once I got home, I emailed Erin with my hilarious experience and wanted to know how her experiment had gone. Although it was in the comfort of her own home, she'd pretty much gone all over herself, too. Nothing like bonding over peeing on yourself!

The moral of the story, though? Even when things don't work

out exactly as you hoped they might, they're worth trying. It may not be what you envisioned. In fact, it may be gross. Really gross. But it may just make for a great—and hilarious—story later!

Don't put your ambitions on hold because you feel too far away from the starting line. There is no time like the present to dive in and get started. So jump in with both feet. Take that cardio class even if your fitness level isn't where you want it to be; you might have to take breaks and modify moves, and that's okay. Start swimming again; it doesn't matter if you feel bikini-ready, just put on a suit and get splashing. Dance; if you have two left feet, it'll just make your moves all the more unique. Bring your sense of humor and simply enjoy the effort.

Most important, find activities that bring you joy. Think back to when you were a kid: what did you love to do? If it's running, great—get out there and pound the pavement. If you had a blast playing softball, join a team—even if you don't know anybody on it, or you're afraid you'll strike out every time. If you loved roller-skating, embrace your inner roller derby queen and grab some skates. Fitness doesn't have to be about the treadmill or weight machines. Do what makes you smile!

Don't limit yourself to activities that feel comfortable and safe. Embrace who you are and be confident in your abilities—or lack thereof. Get out of your comfort zone and don't be afraid to laugh. If you goof, laugh. Make fun of yourself and just be yourself. Trying is half the battle, and perfection is for the birds anyway (assuming that birds are perfect).

Convinced that it's far better to laugh it off? We thought so. Here are some ways to get you laughing, taking yourself less seriously, and feeling happier in 10 minutes flat!

1. **CREATE A HILARIOUS ONLINE VIDEO PLAYLIST.** Seriously, what did we do before YouTube? Life is so much richer—and more hilarious—with online videos. From yelling goats, to dancing cats, to people doing all kinds of humorous things, we love going to the web-o-sphere for a feel-good fix. But instead of just popping online and trying to find something funny to watch when you need a pick-me-up, we suggest creating your own greatest hits video playlist.

   Similar to how you'd make a workout music playlist, this is simply a matter of listing the videos that make you laugh every time you think of them. If you have a YouTube account, you can create a video playlist there, or you can simply open up a blank doc or email and paste links. Either way you do it, set aside 10 minutes to peruse online videos, searching for the ones that really, really tickle your funny bone. (If you need help getting started, we recommend searching for the words *funny* or *hilarious* and then sorting by the view count—normally the ones that have been watched a lot are popular for a reason!)

   It doesn't matter if they're bloopers, improv acts, skits, or animals doing the polka, just choose about ten or so videos that really make you laugh and make a playlist of them. Then, when you're feeling down or need a laugh, you can pull up your personalized playlist and get to cracking up!

(2) **TRY SOME INTERPRETIVE DANCE.** There's no better way to get a good chuckle than by doing something that's a bit cheesy. Something like interpretive dance. For this 10-Minute Fix, all you need is a good sense of humor, some creativity, a timer, and a radio. You can do it with a buddy or by yourself; either way, it's a great time.

Turn the radio to your favorite station. Set the timer for one minute. Then, whatever song is playing, act out the words of the song. So if Katy Perry is singing about fireworks, explode your fingers out as if they were fireworks. Being as silly and as high-energy as possible, interpret the lyrics with your own unique (and, we're confident, awesome) dance moves. When the timer goes off, move the dial to another random radio station for another minute of interpretive dance. (If you get stuck with a commercial, go ahead and interpret that, too!) Do this for a total of 10 minutes, and we guarantee you will be out of breath and having a darn good time.

(3) **REWRITE YOUR CONS AS FUNNY PROS.** If you're like most people, you can easily list your negative characteristics—things you would gladly improve upon in yourself. But have you ever thought about rewriting them so that they were actually more of a (funny) pro than a con—and inspired you to meet a goal?

List a few things about yourself that you think you need to improve, but you're not going to beat yourself up about them. For a positive spin, do two things: (a) find the humor in your negative quirk, and (b) find a tangible way to improve it. A few examples to get you started:

Example 1. *You're too out of shape to be a runner.*

The Bright Side: You've never had to deal with ailments like chafed nipples or shin splints.

The Improvement: If your goal is to be a runner, start incorporating short jogs into your cardio workout routine. You'll be surprised at how quickly you'll be able to build up running endurance. (Just don't do too much too fast to avoid shin splints!)

Example 2. *You can't do more than two real push-ups.*

The Bright Side: No one will ever ask you for help moving heavy furniture.

The Improvement: Practice your push-ups a few minutes every day to improve your strength.

Example 3. *Your office is always a cluttered mess.*

The Bright Side: No one will ever want to use it for their work. Office to yourself!

The Improvement: Take 10 minutes each day to de-clutter.

Get the idea? The point is that we all have weaknesses and character flaws. But we should still try to see the humor and the positive side to our imperfections and use them as an opportunity for reflection and self-improvement. Flip that negative script for the positive.

10-Minute Fixes

LEARN TO LAUGH AT "SCARY" GYM SITUATIONS. Unless you're already a gym rat, the health club can seem like an intimidating place. But we promise that by spending a little time there, you'll see that it's really not. And to get you over the first hurdle of going and getting comfortable, we want you to create a plan of attack at the gym. With a little humor, of course . . .

The worst part about going to the gym is not knowing where to go and which pieces of equipment to use and how to set up that equipment. But having a plan makes it far less scary than just showing up and wandering around, trying to figure out what the heck to do. So here's your plan; it's simple, but commit it to memory for this 10-Minute Fix.

Warm up and scope things out: Locate the stretching area— this is usually marked with mats, medicine balls, and foam rollers. You'll want to first "warm up" there, which means that, yes, you'll do some light stretching. But you'll really use it as a home base to scout out the rest of the gym and get more comfortable. Take note of where the cardio and strength equipment, group exercise room, and any other amenities you might want to check out later are. Note where the towels are for mopping up your sweat and where the paper towels are for wiping down equipment when you're done. Scope out any friendly-looking people who aren't immersed in their earbuds.

Pick a piece of equipment to try: Once you've stretched and scoped, choose from one of the following, which are all gym-newbie friendly and don't require any setting up at all. Bonus points if you can find one next to someone who looks like they could be a bud!

- Elliptical
- Treadmill
- Stair-stepper

Hit the big green button! As soon as you hop on your chosen
piece of equipment, take a breath and just scan the console
for a big green button—it'll usually say "start" or "go." Unless
you're prompted to and aren't allowed to skip it, don't bother
with inputting your gender, age, and weight. Now start moving.
After a few minutes, have fun playing around with some of the
buttons, experimenting with changing the resistance, incline,
and speed where applicable. Chat up the person next to you
about what's on the TV. See it as a cardio adventure—smile!
Stay on for however long you feel like it. Today's victory isn't
about how long you do it but, rather, that you did it!

Cool down—and be proud! Go back to your stretching area,
stretch it out, and be darn proud of yourself for conquering the
gym. Then pick a new piece of equipment to try at your next
visit.

To get even more comfortable with your plan and at the gym,
don't just memorize what you'll do; visualize yourself doing it
naturally and with a sense of humor. See yourself confidently
carrying yourself and laughing off any hiccups. So it takes you a
few minutes to find the button to start the treadmill or you have
to ask someone for help? Who cares? Other members are usually
more than happy to help (and remember a time when they didn't
know how to set up the bike, either), and the staff? Well, you

10-Minute Fixes

pay them to help you, so don't feel silly asking for a little how-to help! You got this, girl!

(5) WORK OUT YOUR FACE. Just like the rest of your body, your face is made up of muscles. Muscles that are in charge of smiling, frowning, and making all kinds of other expressions. While we don't think it's necessary to actually "exercise" these muscles (although that was all the rage in anti-aging in the 80s, and we *highly* recommend checking out a hilarious video of Greer Childers demonstrating this!), we do think it's a really enjoyable way to spend 10 minutes. And it's one heck of a way to have a good time laughing at yourself.

For this 10-Minute Fix, you need access to a mirror. Challenge yourself to a game of How Ridiculous of a Face Can I Make? Then, for five or so minutes (feel free to go longer if you have the time!), try to make the funniest and craziest faces you can. Smush your face up. Elongate it out. Open your eyes wide and stick your tongue out. Impersonate a celebrity or animal— the weirder the better. Consider taking selfies as you go so that you remember—and laugh at—each of them when you're done. Try to pick out the one particular face that was "the most ridiculous." Once done, you can either delete the photos or save them and create a Ridiculous Face Hall of Fame. Looking at this little FBG laugh-at-yourself "memento," as we know from experience, is another great and hilariously awesome pick-me-up. And feel free to play this game with a friend, too.

(6) BECOME YOUR FAVORITE POP STAR. Sometimes one of the best ways to take ourselves less seriously is to actually act like someone else—someone who dances and sings on stage! But don't worry: it's just for 10 minutes and you don't need any singing chops.

First, think about your favorite pop workout tunes. Who is played most on your iPod, exercise session after exercise session? Whoever it is, that's who you're going to become for 10 minutes. (For us, this would be Britney Spears, Gwen Stefani, or Madonna. Who are all, by the way, *awesome* to impersonate for this fix if you're struggling with whom to choose.)

Once you've picked your pop star, put on a few of his or her tunes and then get to doing your best impersonation. Sing along, dance like the person, strut, jump around, thank the crowd—put on a full-out pop star show! Let your imagination run wild as you really embrace the confidence and high-energy of your chosen star. If you happen to have props like a boa, chair, or hairbrush (to sing into, of course!), that can really take things up a notch.

At the end of the 10 minutes, you should be feeling a little silly, but you should also have a smile on your face and have gotten in a nice little workout. Remember, it's all about having a good time and letting go!

(7) **RUN LIKE PHOEBE.** Have you seen that episode of *Friends* where Phoebe runs like a complete maniac and Rachel is embarrassed to be seen with her? If you haven't, Google it. In the end, Rachel discovers that running like a maniac is a blast and feels great. She's forced to embrace her silly side and just enjoy running. We want you to do the same!

Take the next 10 minutes to head outside and run like a fool. It can be in your neighborhood, it can be at a nearby track, it

ENERGIZE!
The Power of Sunshine and Vitamin D

We're so conditioned these days to protect ourselves from the sun that we slather on the sunscreen, don our biggest hats, and cover up from head to toe when we venture outside. But the same sun that blisters our skin also has some benefits, so there's no need to act like a vampire and hide away all the time. Sun exposure kicks off chain reactions in your body that produce vitamin D, which helps the body absorb calcium and keeps your bones strong. Plus, sun has mood-boosting benefits that can help reverse the winter blues (like seasonal affective disorder). No, you can't go throwing on that baby oil and baking in the sun to get a golden tan, but 10 to 15 minutes of sunshine a few times a week will help you meet your vitamin D quota. So get happy in the sun!

can be at a park. It can be with people around or in an otherwise empty field. But be goofy. Flail your arms around. Don't run in a straight line. Heck, take it a step farther and break into a dance when a song comes on that makes you want to dance. Just don't worry what people think or the "right way" to run or dance-run. You're blazing your own crazy trail! (Just look out for the horse.)

The point of this exercise is so you can see that being totally goofy won't kill you. It's to embrace your silliness and make yourself laugh. After doing this, it won't seem so silly to shake your moneymaker in a dance class or hit the weights, will it?

8 **LAUGH IT OUT WITH YOGA.** Ever heard of laughter yoga? Participants laugh their way through class, eschewing traditional yoga poses for gut-busting guffaws of intentional laughter. The idea is that the act of laughing—even if you're faking it—actually boosts health and happiness, including easing the symptoms of depression, migraines, allergies, and asthma.

If you try it yourself, you'll see that fake laughing feels so silly that it will turn into real laughs. Sure, laughter yoga is not equivalent to a full-out sweat session on the treadmill, but there are cardio benefits. So take 10 minutes to do some laughter yoga yourself. Get rid of your inhibitions and belly-laugh. Yes, you will feel silly. But silly is good! Here are a couple "poses" to get you started.

Laughing cow: No, not like the cheese. Get on all fours like you're going to do the traditional cat-cow yoga pose. As you get into cow, belly-laugh "Ha Ha Ha Ha Ha" for five counts as you look toward the sky. As you round your back and reverse the movement into cat pose, change your laugh to a "Ho Ho Ho Ho Ho" for five counts. Repeat this series five times.

Laughing salutation: Start standing, with your hands by your sides. As you walk forward several steps, raise your hands forward in a sweeping motion toward the sky. Reverse the motion as you step backward and end bent at the waist. Match your laugh to the motion; as you walk forward, your laugh goes from low to high. As you walk back, go from high to low.

If you have a hard time conjuring the laughs on your own, check out Laughter Yoga online for guidance. The laughter yoga movement even has a website that can hook you up with events in your area. The site also connects you to great videos of people laughing, and if these genuine laughing fits don't get you laughing, we don't know what will.

10-Minute Fixes

(9) PASS THE HAT OF COMPLIMENTS. We all have things that make us uniquely *us*. Whether it's an amazing natural talent you were born with, a weird learned skill you've perfected over time, or a characteristic you couldn't see yourself without, there is no one in the world quite like you. And now's the time to embrace all of that!

Next time you have a few friends over, do this mood-boosting exercise. It's ideal if everyone knows each other well, but it's totally fine if they don't. Have everyone write each attendee's name on a notecard or slip of paper, along with what they love about that person and what they think makes that person unique. Throw all of the compliments into a hat and take turns reading them out loud. Everybody can save all of their notecards as a mood booster whenever they're feeling down. It's like a mini pep talk from friends for the future!

(10) JOURNAL YOUR ANSWER: *What really makes me happy?* Take 10 minutes to journal about happiness. What really makes you happy? When was the last time you felt happy? Who makes you smile and laugh? Is there any element you'd like to add to your life that would bring you more happiness? What are the activities that bring you joy? What did you love to do as a kid?

After you spend time writing, look at your happiness reflections. How can you go about getting more of that into your life? Being conscious and aware of the activities and people that bring joy to your life will help you live in the moment and try to incorporate those elements more regularly. Take a couple of minutes to schedule some time for those happy-makers, and make it a priority to get them in your life at least once a day!

CHAPTER 10

Love Yo'self, No Matter What

....

There's only one you. And unlike a cat, you have only one life here on earth. And that life is way too short to spend it wishing you looked like an airbrushed celebrity, longing for the abs of fitness models, or beating yourself up for not having chef-like cooking skills, or a perfect home like those you see in glossy magazines and all over social media. The FBGs aren't interested in seeking out perfection but, rather, in embracing ourselves—flaws and all.

We want you to love yourself when you mess up *and* when you succeed. We want you to set realistic goals and expectations for the body you've got. It's part of the reason we're anti-diet and anti-scale: *we're more about enjoying the journey than any specific destination.*

In this chapter, we show you why self-confidence is a must and why the pursuit of perfection does more harm than good. We discuss the negative mental chatter and guilt that are getting in the way of your goals. And we flip the negative thinking to help you embrace your beauty and see all of the positives in yourself. We guide you in the journey to self-acceptance and teach you to treat yourself like a best friend would; that little voice in your head that should be your biggest fan and cheerleader, rather than the opposing team.

Our 10-Minute Fixes in this chapter will help you bust out of the comparison mindset, get rid of guilt that's holding you back, and help you accentuate your positives. We introduce you to confidence-boosting workouts and help you get your self-love back. After all, when you're your most confident, you're also your most beautiful. The more you practice loving yourself, the easier it will become and the more time you can spend rocking what your mama gave you. Life is too short to be anyone but *you*.

A Flawed Idea of Beauty

"Nobody's perfect." We all know this, and yet we beat ourselves up for our lack of perfection. So here is our message to you, and listen up: *Nobody is perfect, and no body is perfect, either.* Everyone can point to her flaws—even those whom we perceive as being flawless. Ask anyone, from supermodels to regular Fit Bottomed Girls, and we are willing to bet that every one of them can name something they'd change. Everyone is her own harshest critic.

Those imperfections, though, are what make us unique. Just think of Cindy Crawford's beauty mark, model Lauren Hutton's gap-toothed grin, or Tina Fey's scar. Those people wouldn't quite be themselves without those signatures.

The definition of beauty changes over time; just head to an art museum and you'll see proof of how much our idea of beauty has shifted across cultures and centuries. Women depicted in art certainly don't seem to fit neatly into today's standard of beauty—imagine

SMOKE, MIRRORS, AND PHOTOSHOP

We briefly mentioned how phony most magazine covers are because celebrities and models are airbrushed within an inch of their lives. This celebrity airbrushing erases inches off of arms and thighs, perfects imagined imperfections, and in doing so gives the consumer unrealistic expectations of what we should look like. We guarantee you'll feel better about yourself when you see the reality that is the Photoshopped celeb.

But don't just take our word for it. We want you to see for yourself, so get thee to a computer. Simply Google "celebrity photoshop" and you will turn up millions of hits of celebrities who have been airbrushed for various magazine covers. We especially recommend searching "celeb photoshop gifs," which flash before and after photos so you can see the transformation.

We understand smoothing a shirt or erasing a blemish for a magazine cover, but obviously this fixing-up has gotten out of hand. They're people, they shouldn't look like dolls! And don't even get us started on how entire arms and fingers go missing. Celebrities and models—hell, *people*—are beautiful enough; we think they're even more so with flaws and wrinkles, rather than with the phony too-smooth skin you often see. So next time you see a celeb looking flawless and you start beating yourself up as a result, remember that looks are oh so deceiving.

seeing Mona Lisa walk the runways at fashion week. And if you think about it, the standard of beauty in the Western world today is really unfair. Professional hair and makeup artists can hide anything, and the right lighting and perfect pose can go a really long way in flattering the imperfect. Where even makeup and lighting fail, airbrushing and technology can accomplish the rest. It's a rare magazine cover that doesn't Photoshop perceived flaws and fix "imperfections." Even though most of us are aware that these types of images are digitally edited, that still doesn't mean we don't compare ourselves to these "ideals" of beauty. It's hard not to, particularly because we're bombarded with these images every day, from billboards to magazine ads to TV commercials. But when even the likes of gorgeous actresses and models have to be Photoshopped to be considered worthy of a cover, what message is it sending to the rest of us?

A Flawed Idea of Body Weight

The media's generalization of thin as the beautiful ideal can also be harmful. It sets us up to believe that there is only one "right" way to look and to be healthy, and that couldn't be further from the truth. There is a wide range of healthy weights, and there is no one-size-fits-all formula. Likewise, believing you should be a certain pant size—especially if the last time you were that size was in toddlerhood—just messes with your mind. Some people will never be a size 6 or 10, no matter how much weight they lose, simply because their bone structure doesn't match that size. Short of some seriously drastic surgery, it's pretty tough to change your bones.

While body mass index (BMI) charts can give you a general range of healthy weights to shoot for, they're not going to be a definitive standard for everyone, either, as they don't account for bone structure or muscle mass. No chart or online quiz is going to give you one specific number that is your perfect weight. We're all individuals, and everyone has her own ideal weight—and even her own range of what will work for her. Use BMI, standards for weight based on your height, and body fat percentage charts as guidelines pointing you in the right direction, not as measures of success or failure. Instead, aim for a body that is strong, flexible, and allows you to do the activities you want to do. Again, not a perfect body according to society, but one that supports the healthy and feel-good lifestyle that you want—and *deserve*.

We're not experts on eating disorders, but they are worth mentioning because media and outside pressures to be thin and beautiful can trigger unhealthy behaviors. While there is no single cause of eating disorders or body dissatisfaction—psychological, behavioral, biological, emotional, interpersonal, and social factors all play a role—research shows that the media do play a part. Studies have linked exposure to the thin ideal projected in the mass media to body dissatisfaction and disordered eating among women. That's why it's so important to make sure you're making changes for the right reasons. Looking fabulous is a great side effect of eating well and working out, but it should never be the sole goal. Rather than focusing your mental energy on that bikini, your dress size, or looking like that cover model, shift your thinking to all of the health benefits you're getting from the good decisions you're making. Concentrate on how balanced your nutrition is, and how much energy you have. A whole-health mentality will keep you focused well beyond swimsuit season.

Beauty isn't just about whether you've got a bikini body or the perfectly applied eyeliner. Beauty really does come from within. Just think of people who don't fit the traditional standard of beauty yet are found extremely attractive by the masses. They typically have a crazy confidence, a swagger, a sense of humor, an amazing talent, a personality that's larger than life. They are imperfect, but they highlight their positives so much that we see their true beauty. Think of that musician you want to make out with when you see him play the guitar or that comedian who is unconventionally pretty in a quirky way. Think of your best gal pals. Do you hang out with them because they're super skinny and hot? Nope. You hang out with them because they're super fun, confident, and a blast to be around. Beauty isn't about looks alone, it's a package deal.

These are some of the reasons we started Fit Bottomed Girls. We wanted women to know that they could be healthy without being a specific number on the scale. They could be fit at a vast range of weights. That there is no one perfect standard because, as humans, we are all so different. We wanted to be a sane voice in all of the incessant chatter to reassure women that they don't need to restrict, or overexercise, or hit a number to be perfect. They're just right as they are. There is beauty in a wide range of looks and most of it comes from within. Like we always say, fit bottoms come in all shapes and sizes!

FIT BOTTOMED MANTRA

"Love yourself first and everything else falls into line. You really have to love yourself to get anything done in this world."

—LUCILLE BALL

The Dark Side of Perfection

Perfection is simply impossible, and aiming for it sets you up for failure before you even begin. That's why we recommend that 80/20 rule—because you need that extra 20 percent of wiggle room. If you aim to have a "perfect" diet, you'll be missing out on a lot of fun and probably unwittingly missing out on nutrients. If you aim to be "perfect" at working out, you'll miss any spontaneous adventure or unplanned sweat session. You'll beat yourself up when you miss a day; you'll feel like a failure. You'll likely give up, because perfection isn't a sustainable place to be.

These reasons are why we're so adamant that it's not about the number on the scale. Things you see as your imperfections don't just disappear when you hit a certain weight or a specific BMI. That magic number won't make your job woes disappear, either. That perfect guy won't automatically land on your doorstep. You may even still have a body part you wish looked different. Losing weight isn't a silver bullet for your life's problems because, when all is said and done, you're still the same person. And it can be super frustrating when you put all of your hopes and dreams on a goal like that, only to find that life isn't all rainbows and bunnies once you reach it.

All of these reasons are why we're so adamant that you must *love yourself.* We're not saying that you should just resign yourself to being the weight or shape that you are now; having goals for self-improvement is a wonderful, motivating, powerful thing. But we want you to set your goals to be smart, healthy, and achievable. Don't keep chasing an ideal in your head that may not be ideal for you. Instead, do the best you can and forget perfection. You don't want to be consumed by an impossible quest—you want to enjoy living. The more time you spend obsessing about how to achieve the impossible, the less time you can spend appreciating who you are and enjoying all the things that make you unique.

So lighten up on the criticism and start accepting yourself as you are. Decide to make changes from a place of love and positivity, not a place of negativity and perfection-seeking. If you're trying your best, let that be good enough and keep trying. Deep down, you know the difference between when you're slacking and when you're working as hard as you can. Let your inner self dole out some tough love when you know that you aren't as focused as you need to be, but don't go too far. A kick in the pants is great; a smack in the head isn't.

It's All About Self-Love

When you're constantly wishing you looked like or acted like someone else, you're discrediting the beautiful and unique person you are right now. When you wish you were someone else, you're telling yourself that you stink. And when you think you stink, it's hard to get motivated to do anything—or feel like you *can* do anything.

Belief in yourself is a must for a happy life. Having this self-confidence and this can't-stop-me-I-rock feeling is essential to getting healthy and being happy. Study after study has shown that when you believe that you can do something—and that you believe that you're worth doing it for—you succeed and can make healthy changes. And when you don't have the belief that you can do it, you are more likely to get tripped up. Without confidence

LOVE YO'SELF, NO MATTER WHAT   239

FROM THE FBGs
The Body Part We Love the Most

FROM ERIN: I won't go into the whole song, but I like my butt; I cannot lie. I know, it seems obvious considering the name Fit Bottomed Girls, but it hasn't always been a tush love affair.

Like most women, I've gone through spells when I wished I could edit my body a bit. Those moments typically occur in a dressing room, when I'm trying on bathing suits in terrible lighting. But I've learned to ignore those moments—they are few and far between unless you live in a dressing room—and embrace the positive. My butt has served me pretty well over the years, after all. It's powered me up hills and up stairs, around bases on the softball field, and up and down basketball courts. It's run around tracks and on treadmills, walked around cities sightseeing. It's heaved itself into toe-touches too numerous to count and added padding to bike seats. It's cushioned falls on the ski slopes and, let's be honest—the sidewalk.

I think my butt looks pretty good in my standard jeans and T-shirt wardrobe, and that matters way more than a poorly lit moment in a dressing room. Plus, my rump is the one place I actually have curves to celebrate. And seriously, what's better than a good butt burn the day after a hard workout?

My butt tends to stay where it should. It tends to fill out my jeans and look decent in yoga pants. And it tends to stay strong to power me through workouts even if it gets twitchy at the end of a lunge-filled sweat session. My butt's not perfect. But it's perfect for me!

you have more negative thoughts about yourself and your ability to reach your goals. This can lead to self-sabotage and going back to past unhealthy behaviors. However, when you start to treat yourself with the love, compassion, and respect that you'd show someone else in your life whom you adored, everything starts to change. Basically, this all boils down to one thing: whatever you think you can or can't do, you're right. So think and believe that you *can* do it!

Now, "loving" yourself doesn't mean stroking your ego until your head is enormous. Instead, it's a quieter and more certain feeling *that you got this*. It's not about proving it to others—it's about proving it to yourself and always having your own back. It's about being open to new experiences and learning. It's about being confident enough to listen to your gut and believe that when the going gets tough, you have what it takes to keep going. *Capiche?*

Cultivating a Healthy Relationship with Yourself

Saying that you want to start talking to yourself like your own best friend is one thing, but how you actually go about doing it is another. And it may seem like a kind of tough, existential thing to change. You might be saying, "Um, ladies? My thoughts are just my thoughts! They just come and go without my permission."

But here's the thing: you can actually shift your internal dialogue from Negative Nelly to Supportive Sally. Sure, it does take practice and time, but the results are way, way worth it. And the first step to getting there is to start to be aware of what thoughts are going through your brain. Don't try to judge them or change them. Just be aware of them and what they're saying.

Now take a deep breath with us and realize that those thoughts are not you. They are the product of years and years of experiences, habitual patterns, and—let's face it—most likely the voice of the naysayers you've had in your life (a not-so-nice boss, parents who weren't supportive, a boyfriend who didn't treat you right, etc.). Again, they are not you. Your thoughts, which many of us are not fully conscious of, are many times like a record that's being played over and over again.

Now, who is really "you"? Well, the real you is the thing/being/ spirit/soul/whatever you want to call it who is watching those thoughts. That's the real you, darling! Not some thought pattern you keep repeating because your mom once told you that you looked heavy in a pair of shorts and then you internalized that as meaning that you should never wear shorts ever again for the rest of your life. No way. The real you is already perfect, glowing, unique, and special. She doesn't need to lose weight, or have bigger boobs, or have straight hair to be lovable. She's beautiful as she is. And she's more than just a body—she's your inner FBG! And she is the one you need to love unconditionally. She's the one you need to check in with daily and identify with. She's the real you. And in support of the real you, you need to begin to call BS on some of those thoughts that aren't supporting her. Or you. You know what we mean.

You still with us? Let's keep going.

After spending a few days watching your thoughts, begin to take note of any limiting beliefs or recurring patterns that you're seeing. Are you constantly comparing yourself to others? Do you beat yourself up when you get dressed? Do you tell yourself you're not good enough? Do the words *fat, stupid,* or *can't* come up a lot?

Awareness is the first step toward being free of heady trash-talk. Then, once you know what thoughts are rattling around in that brain of yours, when you hear them, you consciously interrupt the thought and counter it. Now, don't do it in a mean way—that pretty much defeats the purpose if you bring negativity to it. Instead, remind yourself that you're playing that negative loop, and replace that thought with a nicer, more loving one. Here are a few examples:

Negative repeating thought: I look fat.
Loving replacement thought: I am more than just a body.

Negative repeating thought: I wish I looked like her.
Loving replacement thought: I determine my own self-worth.

Negative repeating thought: I can't do anything right.
Loving replacement thought: I am doing my best.

Negative repeating thought: I hate myself.
Loving replacement thought: I am learning to love myself.

Now, once you have the knack of those down (which may take a few weeks), and your new loving replacement thoughts are more natural, take it up another notch.

Loving replacement thought: I am more than just a body.
Super-loving replacement thought: I love my body as it is.

Loving replacement thought: I determine my own self-worth.
Super-loving replacement thought: I am uniquely beautiful.

Loving replacement thought: I am doing my best.
Super-loving replacement thought: I can do anything that I commit myself to.

Loving replacement thought: I am learning to love myself.

Super-loving replacement thought: I love myself.

It may take time before you fully break the negative thought cycle, but you *can* do it. In fact, those negative thoughts start losing their power the moment you take an active interest in identifying them—and don't let them define you any longer. Instead, you begin to see the world on your terms, focusing on the good and appreciating your body and your unique self. Having these more positive and loving thoughts will help you to feel more comfortable and confident in your skin, which only leads to more good. We know that when we focus on the good and what we like about ourselves, we feel empowered and like we can do anything. And that, our friends, is a healthy and very FBG state of mind.

Drop the Guilt Trip

Of all the negative emotions out there, guilt is one of the worst. Whether it's a result of eating too many slices of pizza, or something more serious like cheating in a relationship or lying to someone, guilt is a heavy, heavy feeling that many get stuck in. Whether the guilty offense is large or small, many of us feel as though we need to punish ourselves and remind ourselves of how terrible we are as penance for said guilty offense. It's as if making one mistake—no matter what it is—should be able to sum up our whole self as wrong, flawed, or downright bad.

Well, part of loving yourself unconditionally is believing that you are not a wrong, flawed, or bad person. Sure, you may make mistakes and do not-so-great things every once in a while (hey, we all do!), but you can't get weighed down by regrets. You need to let yourself off the hook for mistakes that you've made or decisions that you wish you'd made differently; carrying around the burden of guilt and regret won't change what happened, but it will hold you back. You should only hold on to guilt long enough to learn from it. Use it as a springboard to dig deeper into a not-so-positive experience. Why did you do what you did? Is there anything you can learn from it? Was it truly an accident? Examine the deeper causes of the situation you wish you could change, and identify how you could do things differently the next time—then put that into action! Lots of learning and self-discovery can come when you don't just feel guilt, but explore why it's there and then release it.

We'll take you through a really great way to forgive yourself in this chapter's 10-Minute Fixes later, but for now, let's make a point that whenever you feel the tiniest bit of guilt—over saying no to something you don't want to do or telling a white lie—ask yourself what you can learn, and then take a few deep breaths and accept the situation. What happened, happened. Let it go, and move forward stronger, wiser, and more loving from the experience.

A Workout in Self-Acceptance

As you work on accepting yourself for who you are and what your strengths are in the moment, consider choosing workouts that encourage self-acceptance. Not all workouts have this type of philosophy. Pilates and barre classes, for example, call for precision and structure in the movements and alignment—great for mind/body connection, but not as much for freedom of expression. Or look at boot camp workouts—they're structured and regimented. And while super effective and great for discipline, they don't exactly evoke the idea of freedom to be yourself. But some workout genres are geared toward the freedom to express yourself and to accept your flaws and just go with the flow, and we think everyone should have a couple of these types of activities in their workout rotation. Here are a few of our favorites!

- **Zumba:** This hip-shaking Latin-flavored dance class is one of our go-to love-yourself workouts. That's because it's a blast even if you are not so talented in the dance department. It gives enough structure to lead you in getting your groove on, but allows freedom to add your own spin to moves and flare if you've got it. The dance moves allow you to challenge yourself and move your bod in a way that you'll love.

- **Yoga:** The thing we love about yoga is that it's a practice. And that word—*practice*—says a lot. It implies that there is no such thing as yoga perfection. Yoga gets you in tune with your body while letting you try to improve your poses and postures without competition or pressure. Beginners can adapt poses to suit their needs, and there is always room for improvement no matter how long you've been a yogi. Plus, getting in touch with your body and its limits is a good way to embrace your strengths and be more accepting of its weaknesses.

- **intenSati:** We tried out an intenSati workout DVD and fell in love. intenSati combines empowering spoken affirmations with interval training, martial arts, dance, and yoga—a combination you have to do to truly appreciate. It's a sweaty workout that also taps into the mind/body connection, and one of its goals is to heighten your awareness of negative thought patterns—and increase your ability to think positively. It might seem a little cheesy as you're doing it, but it's kind of impossible to walk away from this workout without feeling a little cheerier!

We also love running, walking, and swimming as workouts that are great for cultivating self-acceptance. They can be very meditative, and they allow you to do them how they feel right and best to you. They allow you to both push yourself and to be kind to yourself. No matter what workout you choose, though, always remember you're doing it out of love for yourself, not as a punishment.

Not sure how to put the FBG love yo'self principle into action? Here are easy 10-Minute Fixes to work a little self-loving into your life. And, no, we don't mean *that* kind of self-loving—get your head out of the gutter. (Although, you know, whatever makes you happy.)

1) **BUST OUT OF THE COMPARISON TRAP:** Do you ever look at other people and think they've got it all together while you feel like you're barely treading water? That everyone out there is having more fun and enjoying more success than you are? In these days of social media where everyone is sharing their most awesome successes, it's so easy to get stuck in the comparison trap, comparing everyone else's haves to your have-nots. It's easy to overlook your own awesomeness, so take 10 minutes to bust out of the comparison trap with this quick writing exercise.

Step 1. Look at your life from the outside. Be as objective as you can. Think for a minute about how your life looks to others. Now write a description of yourself as if you were a character in a book or movie. What is this person like? What has she accomplished? What does she do for a living? What does she do for fun? What does she look like? Focus on your successes and try to curb the negative chatter when it crops up.

Step 2: Stay in your objective mindset and write a list of attributes you have that others might admire. How would others describe you? Are you friendly? Funny? Helpful? Kind? Try to keep these positive traits top-of-mind when you start feeling like you're not measuring up.

Step 3: Think back to the last time you felt like you didn't stack up to someone else because of something you saw

on social media. Put on your creative writing cap and conjure up outlandish scenarios as to why things maybe weren't as perfect as they seemed. Did someone's beach vacation get you jealous? Your friend failed to mention food poisoning and getting stung by 92 jellyfish. Does an old high school frenemy have a perfect boyfriend who just brought her flowers? He's actually making up for farting in her presence the night before. It doesn't matter that these scenarios aren't true; it'll still help you realize that not everything is quite as it appears. Remind yourself that for every perfect photo on a social media site, there are probably twenty imperfect retakes. For every bowl of perfect food, there is probably a cluttered countertop that's not being shown. For every adorable baby picture, there is a messy diaper. For every perfect set of abs, there is tons of imperfect sweat to get them.

We tend to see all of our shortcomings and chaos, whereas most people only see you at your best. And others tend to share the achievements and experiences that make them look their best; they're not always in top form. So celebrate your successes and achievements for what they are to you, not how they stack up to everyone else. If you can't get over the mental comparison trap, take a social media break and instead work on living your life rather than watching others and wondering how you compare.

2) **APPRECIATE ALL OF YOUR BODY.** To get you focused on all of the amazing capabilities of your body, work from head to toe and sing your own body's praises. Jot a few words or a sentence or

two for each of these body parts. Concentrate on what that particular part allows you to do and what awesome activities it supports in your daily life. If any negative thoughts pop into your brain, replace them with positive, appreciative ones.

Eyes _____

Mouth _____

Ears _____

Nose _____

Arms _____

Hands _____

Stomach _____

Hips _____

Thighs _____

Butt _____

Calves _____

Ankles _____

Feet _____

When you think of the amazing things your body does on a daily basis and take the time to really appreciate their power, it should make it much harder to be hard on that part—and on yourself. Do this mental exercise any time you're beating yourself—or a particular body part—up, whether it's in the dressing room or when you catch a glimpse of yourself when walking down the sidewalk. Appreciation is the name of the game.

(3) **BECOME YOUR OWN BEST FRIEND.** As cheesy as it sounds, we want you to start being your own best friend. That doesn't mean simply giggling off in a corner by yourself or taking yourself to the movies (although that's part of it!); it means truly supporting

10-Minute Fixes

yourself and treating yourself as a best friend would. Here are a few of our favorite ways to treat ourselves like a BFF—and they only take a couple of minutes each!

Plan a solo outing: You don't need your BFF to do something fun if you're your own bestie—and solo pursuits can be the ultimate in chill-out time. So throw an appointment with yourself into your planner. Then do something nice for yourself with that allotted time—like go to a movie you know your boyfriend or hubby won't want to see, go get a manicure, get a makeover at the makeup counter at the mall, or just enjoy a quiet cup of coffee at your favorite coffee shop. Do an activity purely for the pleasure of it, and enjoy your own company.

Gift yourself: It's so nice when a friend gives you a gift just because it made her think of you. But it's also nice to treat yourself to a special treat now and then just because you're worth it. So spoil yourself once in a while with something fun for no real reason. It doesn't have to be expensive, but make it something you'll really enjoy, like a new book, nail polish, a new piece of workout gear, lip gloss, or a pair of sunglasses.

Check in: You might call your best bud daily to check in or you might be able to go a year without chatting and pick up right where you left off. But don't go that long without checking in with yourself. Whether you vent in a journal about your major stressors or simply meditate to tune in, take just a few minutes to see how you're doing—and give yourself a pat on the back for your recent successes no matter how big or small.

No one can take the place of your best friend, but being your own best bud is a pretty close second. And your relationship with yourself is your most important, so make sure you're making time for you and treating yourself right!

(1) **DRESS YOUR BEST.** Wearing the right clothes for your body can do wonders for your appearance. And when you look good, you feel good, so it's worth taking the time to choose the clothes that will really flatter your body type. Use our quick and easy tips to dress your best—fast!

Step 1: Forget the size obsession. Oftentimes, women try to squeeze into clothing that is too small. Whether it's because they don't want to go up a size or because they've gained a few pounds, it doesn't matter. Wearing clothes that actually fit, no matter what the tag says, is way more slimming and flattering. So cut out the size obsession and don't be afraid to go up to the next size if you need to. It'll be more comfortable and look better, we promise. Besides, because there is no industry standard when it comes to clothing sizes (and some stores implement "vanity sizing"), it shouldn't matter what it says on the tag as long as it makes you feel good! Heck, if it's important to you, use this 10 minutes to cut out the tags altogether.

Step 2: Research clothes for your body type. Whether you're pear-shaped, apple-shaped, or resemble a slice of turkey bacon (no curves to speak of), there is clothing out there that will play up your best features. The right clothing can give curves to the straight-as-an-arrow figure, define waists, and play up good features while minimizing (or maximizing) other areas. If you're pear-shaped (larger on the bottom), think A-line dresses, fuller skirts, and go more fitted on the top. If you carry weight through your middle, you're considered an apple shape. A high-rise pant can control your waist and give definition, while ruffles and cowl-neck options can draw the eye up. If you're slim and want to add curves, think of adding volume, like layers and ruffles on top, flowing skirts on the bottom, and belts.

Step 3: Add your personality. The right accessory can turn a ho-hum outfit into a va-va-va-voom! statement—and it only takes a minute! So invest in a couple of bold pieces you love—a scarf or necklace or cocktail ring can make any outfit special. That way when you have one of those days when you have "nothing to wear" and nothing is fitting quite right, you can spice up your day with an accessory that knocks it out of the park every time.

No matter what you're wearing, you're at your most gorgeous when you're wearing confidence. So throw on that good attitude and get out and conquer the world.

(5) FEEL BEAUTIFUL NO MATTER WHAT. Some days you're not up for the dog-and-pony show that is doing your hair and makeup. But devoting a few minutes to your appearance every day can actually be a really positive experience; it's not vanity, it's a signal to yourself that you matter enough to take care of your body! Whether you're heading to the gym or running an errand, we've got a quick routine that will have you out the door in less than 10 minutes, feeling your best.

Step 1: Throw your hair back into a low ponytail with a funky hair tie, or throw on a decorative headband.

Step 2: Smooth on a combination sunscreen/tinted moisturizer.
This is one of our favorite products, not just for the sun
protection (which is super important) but because it smoothes
the skin and takes almost no effort.

Step 3: Throw on a tinted gloss. A fun lip gloss makes it look like
you made an effort and will moisturize your lips so you're not
tempted to lick them during step class.

Step 4: Curl your eyelashes. Forget the mascara, particularly if
you're heading to sweat in Spin class and don't want that
raccoon look. Instead, simply curl your eyelashes quickly for an
instant eye lift.

Step 5: Smile. If you have no time for any of the above on the way
out the door, this is the most important: Smile! It brightens
up your face no matter how little sleep you got and it lifts your
mood, making you feel beautiful from the inside out.

(6) **WRITE YOURSELF A FORGIVENESS LETTER.** It may seem odd
to write yourself a letter, but this exercise is amazing for breaking down barriers and uncovering unconscious issues that are
holding you back from loving yourself. As discussed earlier,
many times we have guilt or baggage from the past that's holding us back from becoming our best and healthiest. And writing
yourself a forgiveness letter is a great way to let those emotions
go and to help you move on.

To get started, you'll want to find a quiet, peaceful space
that you feel comfortable in and won't be interrupted by others
for the full 10 minutes (or longer if you have the time and want
to keep writing). A comfy chair or a table by a window is a
good choice. Then you'll want to take a piece of paper out (you

10-Minute Fixes

can do this on a computer, but we find that actually writing it down the old-school way is more powerful), and begin your letter like so:

Dear [insert your name],
I love you. And I want you to be the best version of you that you can be. That's why I'm forgiving you for . . .

Then let the words just flow onto the page. Forgive yourself for all of the small and large things in your life that you perceive as mistakes or errors. If you have any baggage you're carrying from failed attempts at getting healthy, drop those. If you've unfairly treated or judged yourself or others, forgive yourself for that, too. Like the journaling exercises, don't feel as if you need to have perfect grammar or even form complete sentences! Just put your truth down on paper.

This is usually a very emotional and charged experience for people, so don't worry if you feel emotional or some tears start to flow (you're alone, so no one will see the ugly cry if you need to go there!). The point here is to bring up your emotions in a safe and loving way, and then to feel them and then release them so that you can get a fresh start. So don't judge what comes up in your letter; just write it down and let it go.

Once you've written your letter, fold it up and then either shred it or burn it (without burning your house down, of course). As you do so, imagine that all of your past worries, negative experiences, and guilt are being brushed away from your past, and that now you are fresh and new. After doing this, you may feel a little tired, but definitely lighter.

If the idea of writing a forgiveness letter to yourself scares you a bit, don't worry. Many of us are afraid to see—or feel—what "might come up" with an exercise like this. But know that because you have that fear, it's probably a sign that there is something inside you that needs releasing. Trust and love yourself enough to know that you'll be safe and secure in this process and that forgiveness is key to moving forward.

And if you ever get stuck beating yourself up about past experiences again, feel free to do this exercise repeatedly. It's great for releasing unmanaged emotions of the past that may be holding you back. Also, if you are harboring resentment toward others, this can be a good way to begin to forgive them. Remember, forgiving isn't forgetting; it's just making the mental room to honor your life now—and not live in the troubles of the past.

(7) **LOVE YOUR PERCEIVED FLAWS.** There seems to be a lot of "problem areas" that the women's publications like to focus on "fixing." But instead of focusing on how we wished these areas looked different on ourselves, what if we all switched our thinking to loving them by using them to our fullest potential? Well, that's exactly what this workout is all about—bringing the love to all the areas of your body!

Warm-up, 1 minute: jumping jacks to love your jiggle. The idea here is to really move your body so that you feel and love all the parts of you that are moving—and especially the parts that are jiggling. Make a point to love the jiggle!

Then do the "Love Yo'Self Circuit." Do each move for one minute. Go through the Love Yo'Self Circuit twice (or more, if you have time) and then cool down.

10-Minute Fixes

10-Minute Fixes

- **Triceps push-ups on the wall to love your wings:** Place your hands on a sturdy wall at shoulder level, standing a couple feet from the wall (if you need to make this easier, stand closer to the wall; if you need to make it harder, stand farther away). Keeping your arms close to your body and keeping your elbows back and not out to the side, lower down so that your face is practically on the wall. Now slowly push yourself out and away from the wall. Repeat as many times as you can in a minute.

- **Side lunge inner-thigh love:** From a standing position, step your right foot out to the side about three feet and keep your left leg straight. Bend your right leg so that you come into a side lunge, making sure that your knee stays in line with your foot. Then push your right leg back and into a standing position again and repeat on your other side. Alternate the sides to work—and send love to—both sides equally.

- **Donkey kicks to kick-start the love to your booty:** From an all-fours position, bring your right knee into your body and then, in a slow and controlled manner, kick your right leg up and out behind you with a bent knee so that you're driving your heel toward the sky. Do 10 kicks with your right leg, and then repeat with the left. Repeat this series until your minute is up!

- **Side plank lifts to love your love handles:** Come into a side-plank position on your forearm with either your legs straight and off the ground (harder—you're just on the sides of your feet) or one leg bent and on the ground (easier—you have some of your weight on the ground). Next, lower your hips straight down to the ground, lightly touching it, and then use your gorgeous obliques to push your hips back up to that side-plank position. Do 10 lifts

ENERGIZE!

Affirmations and Power Songs to Lift You Up!

We love working out with music—it makes you push yourself a little harder, can make you move just a little longer, and it certainly makes working out more enjoyable. We especially love songs that motivate and that incorporate lyrics that can be turned into affirmations that can lift you up even when you don't have your MP3 player connected. Here are a few of our favorites and the mantras they inspire!

"I Will Survive" by Gloria Gaynor. "I will survive" is a great philosophy for any workout!

"Break My Stride" by Matthew Wilder. Nobody's going to hold you down, oh no, "I've got to keep on movin'."

"Fergalicious" by Fergie. Your body will stay vicious too, when you're "up in the gym just workin' on my fitness."

"Hey Ya!" by OutKast. We think everyone should "shake it like a Polaroid picture" at least once a day.

"Bad" by Michael Jackson. "I'm bad, I'm bad, you know it"— and by bad, we mean awesome.

"Push It" by Salt-N-Pepa. "Push It real good"—a mantra that will get you through the end of any tough workout!

"Tubthumping" by Chumbawamba. "I get knocked down, but I get up again, you're never gonna keep me down." An anthem to perseverance if there ever was one!

on one side, and then reverse your side plank so as to work the other side of your body. Repeat this until your minute is up.

Cool-down, 1 minute: Wrap your arms around yourself and give yourself a big ol' hug! Breathe deeply and visualize every area of your body being covered with feel-good love!

10-Minute Fixes

Now, doesn't that feel better than one of those "blast fat" workouts where you do nothing but wish your stomach looked like a model's? We thought so!

8 **PROTECT YOUR WILLPOWER.** Part of loving yourself unconditionally is always making sure that your needs are being met. It also means putting yourself in a position to reach your goals. And a key way to do this is through harnessing your willpower. People talk a lot about wishing that they had more willpower, but the truth is that most of us have about the same amount of willpower as the next person. The trick is all in how we use it.

While most only think willpower is used to avoid unhealthy foods and go to the gym, willpower is actually used anytime you have to do something that you don't want to do. So getting up early to go to work instead of hitting the snooze button ten times? Willpower. Not telling your boss what you *really* think of her? Willpower. Not flipping off a guy who cuts you off in traffic even though you really want to? Willpower, again.

Our willpower is used over and over in a normal day, so is it really any wonder that by the time 6 P.M. rolls around you're not feeling like going to the gym or cooking a healthy dinner? When our willpower is taxed, we're tired, cranky, and want to veg. And then the nonloving, why-can't-I-get-healthy? thoughts start, spiraling us down into a poor-me, nonloving headspace.

So for this 10-Minute Fix, make a plan to protect your willpower so that you can use it to do the things you really want to use it on—making healthy changes and feeling good about it!

Step 1: Take an objective look at your daily routine. From the time you get up until the time you go to bed, make notes of all of the times of the day when you have to force yourself to do things that you don't want to do. Common areas are waking up in the morning, traffic, work projects, relationships, food choices, and workouts you don't like.

Step 2: Pick an area or two that you think you could change for the better. Brainstorm a few ways that you could avoid that situation altogether, make a swap for something less taxing on your willpower, or just make that to-do more enjoyable. Here are some examples:

- **Waking up in the morning:** Go to bed earlier so you're not so tempted to hit snooze or do something in the morning that you love (instead of just rushing to work), so that you're energized to start your day.

- **Traffic:** Commute during different times of the day or begin listening to podcasts or books on CD to better spend the time.

- **Work projects:** Talk to your boss about your workload and possibly delegating any tasks.

- **Relationships:** Make an effort to spend more time with those who leave you feeling good about yourself, and less with those who don't.

- **Food choices:** Avoid walking by the vending machine and pack a healthy lunch so that you're not tempted to make an unhealthy choice or go pick up fast food.

- **Workouts:** Work out in the morning before your day starts to make use of your willpower. Also, choose workouts that you love so that you *want* to do them!

Step 3: Implement your tweaks. Once you have your willpower-protecting tweaks, begin to implement them most days of the week and see if you begin to feel like you have more control and more energy throughout your day. FBGs don't use willpower to love and take care of ourselves; instead we set up our lives in a positive way so that making healthy choices feels good!

(9) **REMEMBER WHEN YOU FELT YOUR BEST.** It's natural for us all to have times in our lives when our self-love has waxed and waned. But for this 10-Minute Fix, tap into a specific moment in your life when you felt your best, your most comfortable in your own skin, and your happiest.

Got your memory? Great! Now think about what elements were there. As you answer each question, really feel the experience and fully put yourself back in that moment.

- Who are you with?
- What are you doing?
- What are you wearing?
- Where are you?
- What emotions are you feeling?
- How do you feel about yourself?
- Are there any other circumstances or factors that contribute to your sense of well-being?

Now, how great would it be for you to get back to that happy time more often? Great, right? So take the next few minutes to see how you can learn from that experience and re-create it more often in your everyday life. Ask yourself the following questions:

- Could you be with those same people again? If not, is there anyone else who makes you feel like they did?
- What other activities bring you that much joy?
- Could you dress like that more often?
- Could you go to that place more often? Or plan for a trip there?
- What other places make you feel that way?
- What other experiences bring you that kind of feeling? How could you do more of them?
- Are there other, more recent times when you felt that same way about yourself?

Loving and taking care of yourself may seem simple, but it's actually influenced in a number of multifaceted and intercon-nected ways. Tapping into a time in your life when you felt loved by yourself and others allows you to see what common elements were there and then allows you to move forward by sticking to more of the stuff that makes you feel good!

(10) **JOURNAL YOUR RESPONSE:** *What I love about myself.* How do I love thee? Let me count the ways! Or, for this journal assign-ment, more like, How do I love me-self? Let me count the ways! Take a full 10 minutes to journal about all the things you love about yourself. From your physical features to your quirks to your

personality traits, everything goes! So just let them pour out. And if you get stuck (many of us feel weird listing off what we love about ourselves because we've been taught not to brag, but, believe us, loving yourself is not being an egomaniac!), try to think of what others who love you in your life would say about you. We bet they'd have lots and lots of amazing things to add to your list!

Conclusion

Whether you're trying to lose weight, get stronger, or maintain the body you have, you need a lifestyle you can get excited about. A *lifestyle* that doesn't deprive you of the things you love or that punishes you for "being bad." Healthy living shouldn't be time-consuming or cumbersome. Figuring out healthy swaps and adding more activity should be a positive, exciting thing. A fun anti-diet thing!

And now that you've seen just how much awesomeness and healthiness you can fit into just 10 minutes, it will encourage you to keep it going. You'll often find that if you did a 10-minute run, you can try for 15 minutes. You'll find that throwing together a healthy meal at home can be faster than heading to the nearest drive-thru. And you'll see that taking 10 minutes here and there to really focus on you and your goals and happiness can really help you get in the right mindset for change. So 10 minutes? That may not sound like a lot, but we hope that you are seeing both immediate and long-term results. You're stacking the building blocks for a tower of healthy habits!

The FBG Lifestyle: Redux

Let's review the 10 main principles of being an FBG:

1. **DITCH THE DIET AND WEIGHT DRAMA.** There is no need to obsess over pounds or count calories—and there are plenty of other ways to measure progress and success. We're no drama llamas, and think you should be, too.

2. **LISTEN TO YOUR HUNGER.** Your body is telling you so much, you just have to listen. Tuning in to your hunger will help you find that happy place between hunger and being too full.

3. **MOVE YOUR BODY.** You don't *have* to be a runner or triathlete to be in shape (although, if you love that, rock it!); if your favorite activity is busting a move in your living room to your favorite pop song, bust your move, girl. And often!

4. **TAKE A BALANCED APPROACH—TO EVERYTHING.** Just as it's important to eat a balanced diet and balance your workouts, take an "everything in moderation" approach to your *life* so that you aren't overstressed, overscheduled, and overwhelmed.

5. **FOCUS ON THE POSITIVES.** Appreciate all of the awesome healthy things you're adding to your life and retrain your brain to turn lemons into lemonade!

6. **GET OUT OF YOUR COMFORT ZONE.** No one likes to be uncomfortable, but it's important to push yourself to stay challenged, set goals, and try new things to keep it fun.

7. **CHILL OUT.** This one is simple: Too much stress bad. Relaxation good.

8. **HELP A SISTER OUT.** Everything is more fun with friends, so don't hoard the healthy fun—spread it like the best virus there is.

9. **LAUGH AT YOURSELF.** Don't take yourself too seriously. Seriously.

10. **LOVE YO'SELF, NO MATTER WHAT.** Accept and love yourself as you are now—flaws and all!

Living each principle on its own is pretty awesome and will help you to be happier and healthier. But put them all together and you've got yourself one amazing FBG-rific life that'll result in a stronger and fitter body, a more confident self, and a life that you've created that you love. All of our principles support one goal: *to feel awesome about yourself from the inside out.* Focus on any of the principles and the accompanying fixes and you'll feel healthier, happier, and better all around. Combine all of them and you'll only gain healthy momentum.

And while we may have given you the steps and the 10-Minute Fixes to help you get there, it's really *you* who has done the life-changing work. You're the one who dug deep and asked yourself the tough questions and found your inner truth and voice. You're the one who did the workouts. You're the one who tweaked your eats to work for you. You're the one who began to see your life through a more loving lens. It's all you, baby! And we couldn't be more proud.

YOUR BONUS 10-MINUTE FIX TO CONTINUE BEING AN FBG FOR LIFE!

We consider our principles of being a Fit Bottomed Girl the basics for getting healthier, as well as good rules for life in general. Whether you've done all of our fixes or just the ones that really spoke to you, we hope they have helped you switch up how you approach living a healthy lifestyle. We know that certain parts of the book will speak to you at different points in time, which is why you can revisit them as often as you like. In fact, consider this a bonus Fix for when you need guidance or hit a rough patch and need to brush up on your FBG principles! Here are just a few situations when you might need to revisit a chapter!

- **Are you obsessing over pounds again?** Revisit Chapter 1 on ditching the diet drama.
- **Are you mindlessly eating past the point of fullness?** Read up on tapping into your true hunger and practice listening to what your body is telling you in Chapter 2.
- **Have you stopped having fun in your workouts?** Find activities you love with the help of Chapter 3.
- **Feeling overscheduled and at your wit's end?** You need to check out Chapter 4 on balance and maybe try a quick fix or two.
- **Feeling like a Debbie Downer?** Peruse Chapter 5 about focusing on the positives—adding in the good rather than seeing anything as deprivation.
- **Hit a plateau and stopped seeing results?** Maybe you need to get out of your comfort zone by setting a new goal with the help of Chapter 6.
- **Stress taking over your life?** Add a few minutes of relaxation to your day with a 10-Minute Fix from Chapter 7.
- **Feeling alone in your fit journey?** Try a couple of our fixes on finding workout buddies and helping others in Chapter 8.

- **Haven't laughed in a week?** You need to get your guffaw on in Chapter 9.
- **Beating yourself up about your imperfections?** Head to Chapter 10 for a dose of self-love!

No matter what the hiccup is on your fit journey, we'll help you to overcome it! And remember: you can *always* visit us online at FitBottomedGirls.com for motivation and tons of support!

Congrats to You, Our Fellow FBG!

We began this book by congratulating you for starting your journey to become a Fit Bottomed Girl. And now we have to *really* congratulate you, because you now know, live, and breathe the 10 principles of living and feeling like a Fit Bottomed Girl. Whether you read the book from start to finish or piecemealed your way through, trying this and tweaking that, we're happy you're here. And we are so very psyched to call you a fellow Fit Bottomed Girl. So, again: Knucks! Sparkle fingers! High five! Woo to the hoo! You have done it!

Now stop reading and go have a blast being a Fit Bottomed Girl—for life!

Additional Materials

Now that you've gotten through the book, we have a few extra materials that will help you along the way. These will help you get started and track your awesome progress.

If you're interested in logging your meals, create your very own food journal, either online or with a notebook. You can log your meals and snacks, when you ate them, how you were feeling when you ate, and how hungry you were before and after. We've included the Hunger and Fullness Scale here again for reference, along with suggestions for how to set up your food journal for success.

Our FBG Shopping List does the thinking for you so you don't get overwhelmed by the grocery store. This comprehensive grocery list includes all of the FBG-approved favorites that are the building blocks of healthy meals. We've even included a few indulgences!

The Two-Week FBG Plan will help you see just how easy it is to take all you've learned and put it into action. We'll help you get started with two full sample weeks of meals and workouts, plus the 10-Minute Fix you should try that day. If you do best with direction, the Two-Week Plan will help you avoid getting lost.

We aren't going to leave you hanging by simply mentioning yummy, healthy meals; we've got the recipes to back them up! Our recipes include a bunch of our quick, easy favorites that don't take a lot of time—or a crazy amount of culinary skill—to make.

Food Journal

A food journal can be a great way to get in touch with your hunger and fullness levels, and to see if you're eating for emotional reasons rather than true hunger. You don't need to count calories in it, but keep track of your food and mood now and then to tune back in to what your body is telling you. Your *hunger level* is how hungry you are before you eat; your *fullness level* is how full you are after your meal or snack. Check out the Hunger and Fullness Scale that follows for a quick reminder. Track your mood, too, noting any emotion you're feeling—whether you were happy, sad, anxious, or bored.

Hunger and Fullness Scale

We talked a lot about listening to your hunger and fullness in Chapter 2, but here's a quick reminder to use as you're filling out your Food Journal. The goal is to eat when you're at about a 3 and stop when you're about a 7.

1 Starving! Will eat anything!

2 Can't stop thinking about how hungry you are.

3 Hungry, with an increased urge to eat.

4 A touch hungry. You could eat a little something, but don't feel like you have to.

5 Neutral. Not really hungry or full.

6 Not very hungry; feels like you still have some food in your stomach.

7 Hunger is gone. Your belly is comfortably full.

8 Those last couple of bites were unnecessary. You've eaten plenty and you know it.

9 Starting to feel uncomfortable. Wish you wore stretchy pants.

10 Thanksgiving Day full, plus. Uncomfortably and maybe painfully full.

FBG Shopping List

Don't know where to begin at the grocery store? Our FBG shopping list will help you separate the junk from the deliciously healthy—and we've even included a few indulgences. The less processed a food is, the better, but remember that nothing is off-limits, particularly if the bulk of your food comes from this list. So go ahead and throw some of our favorite whole foods on your grocery list!

STAPLES

100% whole-wheat bread
Agave syrup
Applesauce (natural, unsweetened)
Brown rice
Coconut oil
Dijon mustard
English muffins, whole wheat
Honey
Jelly (all-natural, low-sugar)
Kashi Go Lean cereal
Marinara (prepared, fewer than 80 calories per ½ cup)
Mayonnaise (low-fat)
Microwave popcorn, 100-calorie mini-bags
Milk (1 percent cow's milk and/or unsweetened almond, coconut, hemp, or soy)
Nut butters (almond, cashew, hazelnut, peanut)
Nuts (unsalted, raw)
Oatmeal (any plain variety—instant, quick oats, or steel-cut)
Olive oil
Olive oil cooking spray
Protein bars (at least 10 grams of protein and less than 5 grams of sugar)
Quinoa
Salsa
Tomatoes (canned, diced)
Tortillas (low-carb, whole-wheat)
Vinegar (balsamic, red wine, and apple cider)
Wasa crackers
Whole-wheat couscous
Whole-wheat pasta

INDULGENCES

Chocolate-covered cherries or strawberries
Chocolate syrup
Dark chocolate (at least 70%, can include dark-chocolate-covered almonds)
Frozen yogurt
Hershey's Kisses

Popsicles

Pringles Minis

Sweetened cereal (Vanilla or
Chocolate Chex)

MEALS IN MINUTES

Frozen healthy entrées (Amy's,
Healthy Choice, Lean Cuisine)

Frozen pizza (American Flatbread,
Amy's)

Frozen soy burgers

Low-sodium broth-based soups

PRODUCE

Apples

Avocados

Bananas

Bell peppers

Berries (fresh and frozen)

Broccoli (fresh and frozen)

Brussels sprouts

Carrots

Celery

Cherry tomatoes

Cucumber

Dried fruits (raisins, cranberries,
cherries, plums, apricots, goji
berries)

Edamame

Grapefruit

Grapes

Jicama

Kale

Mandarin oranges in juice

Mixed greens

Mixed vegetables (frozen)

Onions

Oranges

Pineapple

Red new potatoes

Romaine lettuce

Salad greens, mixed

Scallions

Snap peas

Spinach (prewashed)

Sweet potatoes

White mushrooms

LEAN PROTEINS

Beans (canned)

Boneless, skinless chicken breasts

Canned chunk-light tuna in water

Canned wild Alaskan salmon

Cheese (low-fat cottage cheese,
feta, Parmesan, ricotta, string
cheese, and goat cheese)

Deli meat (nitrate-free, all-natural)

Eggs

Fresh or frozen fish

Greek yogurt (low-fat)

Hummus

Lean beef or bison

Lean ground turkey

Pork tenderloin

Precooked chicken breast slices and
all-natural chicken sausages

Protein powder (low-sugar, non-soy)

Rotisserie chicken

Shrimp (frozen raw)

Tofu

Turkey jerky

Two-Week FBG Plan

Not sure how to *exactly* put all of our workouts, healthy eating tips, and self-love into a day-to-day plan that works for you? Or want to jump-start becoming an FBG? This Two-Week Plan is just for you! With the 10-Minute Fixes that introduce you to how to really live each of the principles, along with balanced suggestions to eat, work out, and chill, follow this plan for two weeks and you'll be living the FBG life like a boss!

Just remember: being an FBG is about respecting your body, so use this as a guideline but listen to your body when it comes to portion sizes and workout intensities. Do what feels right for you! And also remember to hydrate regularly throughout the day.

WEEK ONE

MONDAY

BREAKFAST	MID-MORNING SNACK	LUNCH
Steel-cut oatmeal with a scoop of vanilla protein powder mixed in and topped with blueberries	Low-fat Greek yogurt and an orange	Can of low-fat, low-sodium broth-based veggie soup, plus a small wheat tortilla rolled up with nitrate-free deli turkey slices and avocado slices
AFTERNOON SNACK	**DINNER**	**DAILY TREAT**
Handful of Happy Trails Mix (page 281)	Fish in a Flash (page 282), with side salad and brown rice	Half of a frozen banana smeared with 1 tablespoon peanut butter and drizzled with chocolate syrup

•**Work out like an FBG:** Chapter 3: 10-Minute Fix #3 (Do one of each type of workout from the Try These Cardio, Strength, and Flexibility Plans, page 77), as one master 30-minute workout	•**Take care of yourself like an FBG:** Chapter 1: 10-Minute Fix #2 (Measure Up!, page 24)

TUESDAY

BREAKFAST	MID-MORNING SNACK	LUNCH
Sippable Smoothie (page 283)	Yum Hummus and Veg (page 56)	Big-Ass Salad (page 284)
AFTERNOON SNACK	**DINNER**	**DAILY TREAT**
Low-fat cottage cheese with grapes	Rockin' Rotisserie Chicken (page 55) with Roasted Veggies (page 291) and quinoa seasoned with curry powder, salt, and pepper	Microwaved sweet potato topped with coconut oil and drizzled with agave nectar

•**Work out like an FBG:** Chapter 7: 10-Minute Fix #3 (Do a Yoga Series, page 188) one to three times	•**Take care of yourself like an FBG:** Chapter 1: 10-Minute Fix #8 (Reclaim the Scale, page 30)

WEDNESDAY

BREAKFAST	MID-MORNING SNACK	LUNCH
Low-sugar, high-protein protein bar and fresh berries	Cucumber slices with low-fat Greek yogurt	Grilled chicken sandwich with honey mustard sauce and a side salad with a vinaigrette from fast-food joint or restaurant
AFTERNOON SNACK	**DINNER**	**DAILY TREAT**
Turkey jerky with baby carrots	Big-Ass Salad (page 284)	Punkin' Muffin (page 285)

•**Work out like an FBG:** Chapter 3: 10-Minute Fix #3 (Deck of Cards Workout, page 79)

•**Take care of yourself like an FBG:** Chapter 8: 10-Minute Fix #1 (Transform a Buddy into an FBG, page 203)

THURSDAY

BREAKFAST	MID-MORNING SNACK	LUNCH
Punkin' Muffin (page 285) cut up and mixed with low-fat Greek yogurt and topped with walnuts	Celery with peanut butter	Veggie burger and a sweet potato with coconut oil
AFTERNOON SNACK	**DINNER**	**DAILY TREAT**
Laughing Cow wedge with a tangerine	Brinner That Can't Be Beat (page 286)	Cup of hot cocoa made with 1% milk or unsweetened almond or coconut milk

•**Work out like an FBG:** Off day!

•**Take care of yourself like an FBG:** Chapter 2: 10-Minute Fix #5 (Be Mindful—With Chocolate!, page 48)

FRIDAY

BREAKFAST	MID-MORNING SNACK	LUNCH
Kashi Go Lean cereal with your milk of choice and fresh berries	String cheese with strawberries	Peanut butter and jelly sandwich on whole-wheat bread, plus low-fat Greek yogurt and yellow bell pepper strips
AFTERNOON SNACK	**DINNER**	**DAILY TREAT**
Couple slices of nitrate-free deli turkey topped with avocado slices	Seaweed salad, edamame, and California rolls at sushi restaurant	Apple, chopped and sautéed in a little butter, topped with a small handful of pecans

•**Work out like an FBG:** Walk or run with a friend for 30 minutes	•**Take care of yourself like an FBG:** Chapter 7: 10-Minute Fix #2 (Shower Yourself with Relaxation, page 188)

SATURDAY

BREAKFAST	MID-MORNING SNACK	LUNCH
2 poached eggs with grapefruit	1 ounce of goat cheese with fresh cherries	Gourmet Mini Pizzas (page 287)
AFTERNOON SNACK	**DINNER**	**DAILY TREAT**
Apple with almond butter	Shortcut Soup (page 55)	Square of dark chocolate, smeared with a little almond butter

•**Work out like an FBG:** Chapter 3: 10-Minute Fix #5 (Do TV Workouts, page 88)	•**Take care of yourself like an FBG:** Chapter 4: 10-Minute Fix #7 (Learn Your Portion Basics, page 113)

SUNDAY

BREAKFAST	MID-MORNING SNACK	LUNCH
Sunrise Sammie (page 53)	Turkey jerky with a peach	Shortcut Soup (left over from yesterday)

AFTERNOON SNACK	DINNER	DAILY TREAT
Handful of walnuts and dried goji berries	Fajita Salad (page 288)	Frozen yogurt topped with fresh fruit

•**Work out like an FBG:** Go to a cardio group exercise class, like Zumba or kickboxing	•**Take care of yourself like an FBG:** Chapter 6: 10-Minute Fix #10 (journal entry "Why I want to reach my goals," page 171)

WEEK TWO

MONDAY

BREAKFAST	MID-MORNING SNACK	LUNCH
Steel-cut oatmeal with almond butter and topped with blueberries	Carrots and peanut butter	Big-Ass Salad (page 284)

AFTERNOON SNACK	DINNER	DAILY TREAT
Low-sugar, high-protein protein bar	"Nacho" Unhealthy Nachos (page 289)	Handful of chocolate-covered cherries or strawberries

•**Work out like an FBG:** Chapter 6: 10-Minute Fix #7 (Flexibility Workout: Stability Ball Stretch, page 168)	•**Take care of yourself like an FBG:** Chapter 7: 10-Minute Fix #7 (Get a Better Night's Sleep, page 191)

TUESDAY

BREAKFAST	MID-MORNING SNACK	LUNCH
Sippable Smoothie (page 283)	String cheese with two apricots	Turkey or bison burger and a baked potato topped with salsa

AFTERNOON SNACK	DINNER	DAILY TREAT
Yum Hummus and Veg (page 56)	Two soft chicken tacos with avocado and lots of salsa, side of refried beans, from a Mexican restaurant	Chocolate-Avocado Mousse (page 290)

•Work out like an FBG: Chapter 3: 10-Minute Fix #3 (Try These Cardio, Strength, and Flexibility Plans, Strength: Five Minutes to the Burn, page 80); repeat 2–3 times if you have time and the energy!	•Take care of yourself like an FBG: Chapter 5: 10-Minute Fix #7 (Set Up a Gratitude Email or Text Exchange, page 136)

WEDNESDAY

BREAKFAST	MID-MORNING SNACK	LUNCH
2 eggs scrambled with spinach and topped with feta	Handful of cashews and dried unsweetened cranberries	Tandoori chicken with vegetarian curry and a little rice from an Indian restaurant

AFTERNOON SNACK	DINNER	DAILY TREAT
Jicama strips and a hard-boiled egg	Rockin' Rotisserie Chicken (page 55) with Kale Chips (page 290) and brown rice	Funky Monkey Smoothie (page 291)

•Work out like an FBG: Off day!	•Take care of yourself like an FBG: Chapter 9: 10-Minute Fix #6 (Become Your Favorite Pop Star, page 226)

THURSDAY

BREAKFAST	MID-MORNING SNACK	LUNCH
½ cup of cottage cheese with a whole-wheat English muffin topped with peanut butter	Kale Chips (left over from last night's dinner) with fresh cherries	Can of tuna mixed with low-fat mayo on whole-grain crackers and a side salad

AFTERNOON SNACK	DINNER	DAILY TREAT
Applesauce mixed with almond butter	Big-Ass Salad (page 284)	Low-fat ricotta cheese topped with cocoa powder and agave syrup

•**Work out like an FBG:** Chapter 5: 10-Minute Fix #5 (Do Your Workouts with Affirmations, page 134)	•**Take care of yourself like an FBG:** Chapter 7: 10-Minute Fix #5 (Try a Self-Massage, page 190)

FRIDAY

BREAKFAST	MID-MORNING SNACK	LUNCH
Parfait of alternating layers of low-fat Greek yogurt, berries, and walnuts, drizzled with honey	Popcorn with mixed nuts	Cup of tomato soup and a grilled cheese sandwich

AFTERNOON SNACK	DINNER	DAILY TREAT
Red pepper slices with low-fat Greek yogurt	Handful of chips with salsa, and a taco salad ordered without the shell with grilled chicken and salsa as dressing, from a Mexican restaurant	Handful of chocolate chips, almonds, and dried cranberries

•**Work out like an FBG:** Chapter 3: 10-Minute Fix #3 (Try These Cardio, Strength, and Flexibility Plans, Strength Workout: Short Circuit, page 78)	•**Take care of yourself like an FBG:** Chapter 10: 10-Minute Fix #1 (Bust Out of the Comparison Trap, page 247)

SATURDAY

BREAKFAST	MID-MORNING SNACK	LUNCH
Sautéed kale, topped with dried cranberries and 1 sliced chicken sausage link	Couple slices of nitrate-free deli roasted chicken topped with avocado slices	Turkey sub sandwich with apple slices

AFTERNOON SNACK	DINNER	DAILY TREAT
Microwaved sweet potato topped with a little olive oil, salt, and pepper	Fish in a Flash (page 282), with a veggie of choice and quinoa	Scoop of frozen yogurt, sprinkled with peanuts

•**Work out like an FBG:** Chapter 6: 10-Minute Fix #7 (Push-Yourself Workouts, Cardio Workout: Striders, page 166)

•**Take care of yourself like an FBG:** Chapter 2: 10-Minute Fix #1 (Distract and Delay Before You Dish Up, page 45)

SUNDAY

BREAKFAST	MID-MORNING SNACK	LUNCH
Whole-wheat tortilla filled with 2 scrambled eggs, salsa, and cilantro	Grape tomatoes and a hard-boiled egg	Whole-wheat pita filled with diced chicken, grapes, romaine lettuce, and a dollop of low-fat Greek yogurt

AFTERNOON SNACK	DINNER	DAILY TREAT
1 cup of low-sodium chicken soup	Gourmet Mini Pizzas (page 287)	Chocolate-covered cherries

•**Work out like an FBG:** Do a yoga or Pilates workout DVD

•**Take care of yourself like an FBG:** Chapter 9: 10-Minute Fix #10 (journal entry "What really makes me happy?" page 230)

Recipes

We FBGs love to eat! And whether you love to cook or not, it's important to have some quick, yummy, and simple go-to recipes on hand so that no matter how your day goes, you have good eats to whip up. Most of these recipes are written to provide one or two servings, but it's easy to feed a larger crowd with them—just double, triple, or quadruple them!

HAPPY TRAILS MIX

Serves 1

Not just for the hikers among us, trail mix can be a great way to get some healthy fats and cure a hankering for sweets, with its sweet-and-salty mix of goodies. Watch your portions and pay attention to your hunger cues, as it doesn't take long for this filling snack to satisfy.

1 tablespoon your favorite unsalted nuts (cashews, almonds, peanuts, etc.)

1 tablespoon unsweetened dried fruits (raisins, cranberries, pineapple, cherries, etc.)

1 teaspoon unsalted seeds (pumpkin, sunflower, etc.)

1 teaspoon dark chocolate chips (optional)

1. Combine all the ingredients in a baggie or reusable container and eat!

FISH IN A FLASH

Serves 2

Fish is an awesome source of protein and can be cooked quickly and easily under the broiler with just a little bit of olive oil—— even when it's frozen! So always keep a stash in your freezer so that you can make this dish anytime. Steam some frozen veggies and a helping of quick-cooking brown rice, and you're all set.

1 pound frozen fillets of white fish (like tilapia, cod, or sole)

1 tablespoon olive oil

Salt and pepper to taste

2 lemon wedges

1. Preheat the broiler to medium-high heat.

2. Rinse the fish fillets under cold water and pat dry with a clean paper towel. Brush each side of the fish with olive oil. Sprinkle with salt and pepper, and place on a baking sheet lined with foil.

3. Broil for 12 to 15 minutes or until the fish flakes easily with a fork and is opaque in the center. (You shouldn't need to flip the fish at all unless your fillets are very thick.)

4. Serve with lemon wedges and enjoy!

SIPPABLE SMOOTHIE

Serves 1

We usually say to eat your calories rather than drink them, but a smoothie is a good option for those who just don't like to eat in the morning or who need a quick snack on the go. You can even throw the ingredients in a blender and then in the fridge the night before to save time.

1 cup washed and trimmed fresh spinach or kale

½ cup frozen berries of your choice (we like a mix of blueberries and strawberries best)

¼ medium banana, peeled

1 tablespoon almond butter

1 scoop of your favorite protein powder

1 cup unsweetened coconut or almond milk

1. Combine all the ingredients in a blender and blend until smooth. If too thick, add a little cold water. If too thin, add a few ice cubes. Sip and enjoy!

BIG-ASS SALAD

Serves 1

Not to brag, but we can make a mean salad. Like a salad the size of your face. Or your small pet. A gloriously enormous salad that can be described no other way but as a Big-Ass Salad. And, boy, does it fill you up and, man oh man, does it make you feel good!

3 cups baby spinach leaves

1 cup mixture of your favorite veggies: chopped broccoli, cauliflower, cabbage, jicama, radishes, cucumber, celery, zucchini

½ cup chopped red, orange, or yellow bell pepper strips

½ cup cherry tomatoes

¼ cup broccoli or alfalfa sprouts

½ cup chopped pieces of your favorite fruit (apple, grapefruit, mango, etc.)

¼ cup of your favorite nuts or seeds (almonds, sunflower seeds, pecans, cashews, walnuts, pumpkin seeds)

Big-Ass Salad Dressing (page 287) or your favorite

4 ounces your favorite cooked protein (salmon, turkey, chicken, tempeh, etc.)

1 tablespoon crumbled goat cheese or feta

Freshly cracked black pepper to taste

1. In a very large bowl (a mixing bowl works best), combine the spinach, veggie of choice, bell pepper, tomatoes, sprouts, fruit, and nuts. Drizzle with the dressing. Mix thoroughly with tongs.

2. Top the salad with the protein of choice, the cheese, and the pepper. Get your Big-Ass-Salad-eating on!

BIG-ASS SALAD DRESSING

Serves 1

This single-serving recipe gives you quite a bit of dressing to use so that every leaf and chopped veggie of your salad is covered but it's not drowning in dressing. The only downside of this dressing is that you need to eat it pretty much as soon as you make it—but that just proves its freshness!

1 orange, peeled and broken into sections
1 tablespoon rice wine vinegar or apple cider vinegar
1 tablespoon almond butter

1. Place the ingredients in a blender and blend until smooth and creamy!

PUNKIN' MUFFIN

Serves 12 (two mini-muffins per serving)

This easy-to-make muffin is an FBG fave. And while it may not be totally balanced, it's so simple and is the perfect option when you get an afternoon hankering for a sweet treat. If you'd like these to pack a protein punch, mix a serving of protein powder with two tablespoons of milk for a frosting, and you'll have a nutritional profile you can feel good about.

Nonstick cooking spray

15-ounce can unsweetened pureed pumpkin

Box of spice cake mix or chocolate cake mix

1. Preheat the oven to 400 degrees. Spray a mini-muffin baking tin with nonstick cooking spray.

2. Combine the pumpkin puree with the cake mix until smooth.

3. Drop the batter into the mini-muffin cups and bake for 20 minutes. Muffins are done when a toothpick inserted comes out clean.

4. Cool on a baking rack and enjoy!

BRINNER THAT CAN'T BE BEAT

Serves 1

Breakfast for dinner, or brinner, can be a fast feast. And this is one of Jenn's favorites! Filling, high in protein, packed with veggies—this scramble is a winner any time of day. Serve it with a microwaved sweet potato topped with a teaspoon of coconut oil and a dash of salt, and you're good to go!

½ tablespoon olive oil

½ bell pepper, chopped

2 ounces nitrate-free smoked turkey or roasted chicken

1 cup spinach leaves

½ cup egg whites (about 4–5 egg whites)

1 tablespoon softened goat cheese

Salt and pepper to taste

Sriracha or other hot sauce (optional)

1. In a medium skillet over medium heat, heat the olive oil. Add the bell pepper and cook for 4 minutes. Add the turkey and spinach, and cook until the spinach is wilted, about 1 minute.

2. Add the egg whites and scramble with the bell pepper and meat. Continue cooking until the whites are solid, another 3 to 4 minutes.

3. Transfer to a plate, and top with the goat cheese, salt, pepper, and hot sauce.

GOURMET MINI PIZZAS

Serves 1

Make-your-own pizzas are a much healthier option than bringing a frozen one home from the grocery store. And they can let you get really creative in the kitchen—there's no shortage of topping ideas and combinations to try! Grab a side salad, a piece of fruit for dessert, and you've got a homemade pizza meal—fast.

1 whole-wheat English muffin, halved

2 tablespoons low-sodium pizza or tomato sauce

¼ cup of your favorite veggies

¼ cup of your favorite protein (beans, chicken, turkey, etc.)

¼ cup shredded or crumbled mozzarella, goat, feta, or blue cheese

1. Place the muffin halves on a heatproof plate. Top evenly with the tomato sauce, then sprinkle on the veggies, protein, and cheese. Pop in the toaster oven or in a 350-degree oven until the cheese has melted. Pizza party!

FAJITA SALAD

Serves 1

Sliced pre-cooked chicken breasts sold at many grocery stores make this meal a snap! And all of the fun toppings turn this salad into a full-out fiesta. A super-filling and healthy fiesta at that!

½ tablespoon coconut oil
½ red bell pepper, sliced
¼ medium onion, sliced
1 garlic clove
½ tablespoon fajita seasoning
4 ounces pre-cooked sliced chicken breast, diced
4 cups mixed salad greens
2 tablespoons guacamole
¼ cup salsa
2 tablespoons shredded low-fat cheese
2 tablespoons minced jalapeño (optional)

1. In a medium skillet over medium-high heat, heat the oil and sauté the bell pepper, onion, and garlic until soft and slightly blackened, about 3 minutes.

2. Remove the veggies from the pan and transfer to a small bowl. Add the fajita seasoning and chicken breast, and stir.

3. Place the salad greens in a large bowl. Top with the chicken-and-veggie mixture and toss.

4. Dress the salad with the guacamole and salsa, and top with the cheese and jalapeño. Have a party in your mouth. ¡Olé!

"NACHO" UNHEALTHY NACHOS

Serves 1

Instead of hitting the drive-thru for greasy Mexican food, serve up your own nachos at home with way fewer calories and fat— and much more nutrition! With these nachos you can set out tons of healthy ingredients and pile on your favorites.

2 cups baked tortilla chips
2 tablespoons shredded low-fat cheddar cheese
3 cups mixed greens
½ cup drained canned black beans
1 cup toppings of your choice: onions, tomatoes, black olives, avocado, cilantro, jalapeños, etc.
¼ cup of your favorite salsa

1. Place the tortilla chips on a large miocrowave-safe plate. Cover with the cheese and place in microwave until cheese is melted.

2. Pile on the greens, beans, and other toppings. Drizzle with you favorite salsa, and get to crunchin'!

CHOCOLATE-AVOCADO MOUSSE

Serves 2

This three-ingredient mousse is downright life-changing. Seriously.

1 ripe banana
1 ripe avocado, peeled and pitted
2 tablespoons unsweetened cocoa powder

1. Combine the ingredients in a blender or food processor. Blend until smooth, creamy, and oh so delicious!

KALE CHIPS

Serves 2

You've probably heard about these before—and with good reason. They're addictively crunchy and make for a satisfying snack that is good for you!

1 bunch kale
½ tablespoon olive oil
Cajun seasoning (like Slap Ya Mama)

1. Preheat the oven to 350 degrees.

2. Cut the stems away from the leaves of the kale and discard. Toss the kale leaves with the olive oil and seasoning.

3. Spread the seasoned kale leaves on a parchment paper–lined cookie sheet and bake for 10 to 12 minutes or until crunchy.

FUNKY MONKEY SMOOTHIE

Serves 1

Oh, it's time to get funky! This chocolate-peanut-banana smoothie is sure to have you swinging from the trees, because it's a tasty and nutritious way to get a chocolate–peanut butter fix!

½ a frozen peeled banana
1 tablespoon peanut butter
1 scoop chocolate protein powder
1 cup low-fat milk or unsweetened coconut or
   almond milk

1. Combine the ingredients in a blender until smooth. And awesomely funky, obviously.

ROASTED VEGGIES

Serves 2

It is simply ah-mazing what some olive oil, salt and pepper, and time in an oven can do for veggies. Pretty much any veggie you can put on a pan in the oven becomes delicious this way.

2 cups of your favorite cut-up veggies (Brussels sprouts,
   broccoli slaw, jicama, zucchini, yellow squash, bell peppers,
   onions, etc.)
1 tablespoon olive oil
Salt and pepper

1. Preheat the oven to 400 degrees.

2. Spread the veggies evenly on a baking sheet. Drizzle with the olive oil and sprinkle liberally with salt and pepper. Roast until the veggies are tender and browned, 12 to 18 minutes, depending on the thickness of the vegetable. Stir occasionally as the veggies roast.

Notes and Sources

Introduction

"How to Lift Your Mood? Try Smiling." *Time.*
http://www.time.com/time/health/article/0,8599,1871687,00.html

"Can Smiling Make You Happy?" *Research and Teaching Showcase.*
http://web.psych.ualberta.ca/~varn/bc/Kleinke.htm

"Smile: A Powerful Tool." *Psychology Today.*
http://www.psychologytoday.com/blog/prefrontal-nudity/201207/smile-
powerful-tool

"Grin and Bear It: Smiling Facilitates Stress Recovery." *Science Daily.*
http://www.sciencedaily.com/releases/2012/07/120730150113.htm

Chapter 1

"Dieting Linked to Weaker Immune System." *About.com.*
http://sportsmedicine.about.com/od/sportsnutrition/a/060304.htm

"How Crash Diets Harm Your Health." *CNN.*
http://www.cnn.com/2010/HEALTH/04/20/crash.diets.harm.health/index
.html)

"Crash Dieting 'Makes You Thick.'" *BBC.*
http://news.bbc.co.uk/2/hi/sci/tech/specials/sheffield_99/448788.stm

"Weight Loss Can Be Contagious, Study Suggests." *Science Daily.*
http://www.sciencedaily.com/releases/2012/02/120214122124.htm

"Phys Ed: Does Music Make You Exercise Harder?" *New York Times.*
http://well.blogs.nytimes.com/2010/08/25/phys-ed-does-music-make-you-exercise-harder/

The President's Challenge Adult Fitness Test.
http://www.adultfitnesstest.org/testInstructions/muscularStrengthAnd
Endurance/halfSitups.aspx;
http://www.adultfitnesstest.org/testInstructions/
muscularStrengthAndEndurance/pushups.aspx;
http://www.adultfitnesstest.org/testInstructions/flexibility/sitandreach.aspx

"The Health Benefits of Journaling." *Psych Central.*
http://psychcentral.com/lib/2006/the-health-benefits-of-journaling/

Chapter 2
"Overeating: Understanding and Taking Back Control." *This Emotional Life,* PBS.
http://www.pbs.org/thisemotionallife/blogs/overeating-understanding-and-taking-back-control

"Addicted to Food? How to Break Your Habit." *Today.*
http://today.msnbc.msn.com/id/12934360/ns/today-today_health/t/addicted-food-how-break-your-habit/#.UPLqsG_O0bg

"Could Drinking Water Before Meals Help You Lose Weight?" *Womenshealth .gov.*
http://www.womenshealth.gov/news/headlines/642324.cfm

"It Could Be Old Age, or It Could Be Low B_{12}." *New York Times.*
http://www.nytimes.com/2011/11/29/health/vitamin-b12-deficiency-can-cause-symptoms-that-mimic-aging.html?_r=0

"Vitamin B_{12}." *MedlinePlus.*
http://www.nlm.nih.gov/medlineplus/ency/article/002403.htm

"Iron." Office of Dietary Supplements, *National Institutes of Health.*
http://ods.od.nih.gov/factsheets/Iron-HealthProfessional/

Chapter 3
"American Heart Association Recommendations for Physical Activity in
Adults." *American Heart Association.*
http://www.heart.org/HEARTORG/GettingHealthy/PhysicalActivity/
StartWalking/American-Heart-Association-Guidelines_UCM_307976_Article
.jsp

"The 10-Minute Workout, Times Three." *New York Times.*
http://well.blogs.nytimes.com/2012/07/25/the-10-minute-workout-times-three/

"Exercise for Depression: How It Helps." *WebMD.*
http://www.webmd.com/depression/features/does-exercise-help-depression

"Exercise and Chronic Disease: Get the Facts." *Mayo Clinic.*
http://www.mayoclinic.com/health/exercise-and-chronic-disease/MY02165

"Study Finds Exercise Adds to Life Expectancy, Even for Obese." *Los Angeles
Times.*
http://articles.latimes.com/2012/nov/07/science/la-sci-exercise-obese-20121107

"Exercise: 7 Benefits of Regular Physical Activity." *Mayo Clinic.*
http://www.mayoclinic.com/health/exercise/HQ01676

"Exercise Helps You Sleep." *WebMD.*
http://www.webmd.com/sleep-disorders/news/20100917/exercise-helps-you-
sleep

"Exercise for Good Sex." *Psychology Today.*
http://www.psychologytoday.com/blog/exercise-and-mood/201203/exercise-
good-sex

"7 Ways Exercise Can Improve Your Sex Life." *Fitbie.*
http://fitbie.msn.com/get-fit/tips/7-ways-exercise-can-improve-your-sex-life

"7 Mind-Blowing Benefits of Exercise." *U.S. News & World Report.*
http://health.usnews.com/health-news/diet-fitness/slideshows/7-mind-blowing-
benefits-of-exercise

"Kick It Up With Cardio Exercise." *WebMD.*
http://www.webmd.com/fitness-exercise/guide/kick-up-with-cardio-exercise

"Flexible Benefits." *American Council on Exercise.*
http://www.acefitness.org/acefit/fitness-fact-article/30/flexible-benefits/#sthash
.u5bBCkO2.dpbs

"Healthy Hydration." *American Council on Exercise.*
http://www.acefitness.org/acefit/fitness-fact-article/173/healthy-hydration/

"The Rest Is Easy." *Runner's World.*
http://www.runnersworld.com/running-tips/rest-easy

"7 Benefits of Circuit Training (and One Downside)." *Shape.*
http://www.shape.com/fitness/workouts/7-benefits-circuit-training-and-one-
downside

"Perceived Exertion (Borg Rating of Perceived Exertion Scale)." *Centers for
Disease Control and Prevention.*
http://www.cdc.gov/physicalactivity/everyone/measuring/exertion.html

"Monitoring Exercise Intensity Using Perceived Exertion." *American Council on
Exercise.*
http://www.acefitness.org/acefit/fitness-fact-article/48/monitoring-exercise-
intensity-using-perceived/

"What Is High Intensity Interval Training (HIIT) and What Are the Benefits?"
American Council on Exercise.
http://www.acefitness.org/acefit/expert-insight-article/3/104/what-is-high-
intensity-interval-training-hiit/

"Pulse." *MedlinePlus.*
http://www.nlm.nih.gov/medlineplus/ency/article/003399.htm

"Target Heart Rate and Estimated Maximum Heart Rate." *Centers for Disease
Control and Prevention.*
http://www.cdc.gov/physicalactivity/everyone/measuring/heartrate.html

Chapter 5

"Talk Yourself Fit." *Prevention*.
http://www.prevention.com/fitness/fitness-tips/certain-sentences-can-improve-muscle-strength

"Positive Shrinking: Writing About the Things That Mean Most Can Help Us Lose Weight." *The Daily Mail*.
http://www.dailymail.co.uk/news/article-2083348/Positive-shrinking-Writing-things-mean-help-lose-weight.html

"A Serving of Gratitude May Save the Day." *New York Times*.
http://www.nytimes.com/2011/11/22/science/a-serving-of-gratitude-brings-healthy-dividends.html?_r=0

"Positive Thinking: Reduce Stress by Eliminating Negative Self-Talk." *Mayo Clinic*.
http://www.mayoclinic.com/health/positive-thinking/SR00009

"Fruits and Veggies to Buy Organic." *Prevention*.
http://www.prevention.com/food/healthy-eating-tips/fruits-and-veggies-buy-organic

"Unraveling the Sun's Role in Depression." *WebMD*.
http://www.webmd.com/mental-health/news/20021205/unraveling-suns-role-in-depression

Chapter 6

"Sticking With Smaller Goals Keeps Weight Loss on Track." *ScienceDaily*.
http://www.sciencedaily.com/releases/2013/01/130117132931.htm

"Helping Athletes Go for the Gold." *Psychology Today*.
http://www.psychologytoday.com/articles/199905/helping-athletes-go-the-gold

Brainy Quote.
http://www.brainyquote.com/quotes/topics/topic_motivational.html#DFhMdFFxyVuo09Ul.99

Chapter 7

"Coping With Excessive Sleepiness: Will better sleep help you avoid extra pounds?" WebMD
http://www.webmd.com/sleep-disorders/excessive-sleepiness-10/lack-of-sleep-weight-gain

"Can Stress Cause Weight Gain?" *WebMD*
http://www.webmd.com/diet/features/can-stress-cause-weight-gain

"Brief Diversions Vastly Improve Focus, Researchers Find." *Science Daily.*
http://www.sciencedaily.com/releases/2011/02/110208131529.htm

"13 Foods That Fight Stress." *Prevention.*
http://www.prevention.com/mind-body/emotional-health/healthy-foods-reduce-stress-and-depression

"8 Foods That Fight Stress." *Woman's Day.*
http://www.womansday.com/health-fitness/stress-management/8-foods-that-fight-stress-103870#slide-2

"Exercise and stress: Get moving to manage stress." *Mayo Clinic.*
http://www.mayoclinic.com/health/exercise-and-stress/SR00036

"Yoga for Stress Management." *WebMD.*
http://www.webmd.com/fitness-exercise/features/yoga-for-stress-management

"When Exercise Stresses You Out." *New York Times.*
http://well.blogs.nytimes.com/2013/03/13/when-exercise-stresses-you-out/

"Coffee Promotes Cortisol Production and Weight Gain." NaturalNews.com
http://www.naturalnews.com/034674_coffee_cortisol_weight_gain.html

"Bad Mood, Low Energy? There Might Be a Simple Explanation."
http://healthland.time.com/2012/01/19/bad-mood-low-energy-there-might-be-a-simple-explanation/

"Caffeine content for coffee, tea, soda and more." *Mayo Clinic.*
http://www.mayoclinic.com/health/caffeine/AN01211

"Health Benefits of Green Tea." *WebMD.*
http://www.webmd.com/food-recipes/features/health-benefits-of-green-tea

"5 Ways Sleeping Less Makes You Gain Weight." *Prevention.*
http://www.prevention.com/weight-loss/weight-loss-tips/how-lack-sleep-makes-you-gain-weight

"9 Surprising Reasons to Get More Sleep." *WebMD.*
http://www.webmd.com/sleep-disorders/features/9-reasons-to-sleep-more

Good Reads.
http://www.goodreads.com/quotes/11924-the-time-to-relax-is-when-you-don-t-have-time

"Sleep Hygiene Tips." *Centers for Disease Control and Prevention.*
http://www.cdc.gov/sleep/about_sleep/sleep_hygiene.htm

"Evidence Builds That Meditation Strengthens the Brain." *Science Daily.*
http://www.sciencedaily.com/releases/2012/03/120314170647.htm

"Mindful Multitasking: Meditation First Can Calm Stress, Aid Concentration." *Science Daily.*
http://www.sciencedaily.com/releases/2012/06/120614094118.htm

"Mindfulness Intervention for Stress Eating to Reduce Cortisol and Abdominal Fat among Overweight and Obese Women: An Exploratory Randomized Controlled Study." *Journal of Obesity.*
http://www.hindawi.com/journals/jobes/2011/651936/

"Studies Show Benefits of Controlled Breathing to Mind and Body." *Southern Methodist University NewsCenter.*
http://smu.edu/experts/pitches/breathing-research.asp

"The Best Way to Breathe." *Discovery Fit & Health.*
http://health.howstuffworks.com/wellness/stress-management/the-best-way-to-breathe.htm

"Breath of Relief." *CBS New York.*
http://newyork.cbslocal.com/2012/04/05/seen-at-11-breath-of-relief/

Chapter 8

"Obesity spreads to friends, study concludes." *New York Times*.
http://www.nytimes.com/2007/07/25/health/25iht-fat.4.6830240.html?page
wanted=all&_r=1&

"It Actually Is Better (and Healthier) to Give Than to Receive, Study Finds."
Science Daily.
http://www.sciencedaily.com/releases/2013/02/130204184300.htm

"Burning More Calories Is Easier When Working out With Someone You
Perceive as Better." *Science Daily*.
http://www.sciencedaily.com/releases/2012/11/121126130938.htm

"Do Good, Feel Good." *MSN Healthy Living*.
http://healthyliving.msn.com/diseases/depression/do-good-feel-good-1

"How to Be Happier Today." *Inc.*
http://www.inc.com/jessica-stillman/happiness-its-easier-than-you-think.html

"Don't Throw Out Those Used Sneaks! How to Recycle Old Fitness Gear."
FitSugar.
http://www.fitsugar.com/How-Recycle-Old-Running-Shoes-2989309

Chapter 9

"Scientists Hint at Why Laughter Feels So Good." *New York Times*.
http://www.nytimes.com/2011/09/14/science/14laughter.html?_r=0

"Laughter Yoga, Serious Benefits." *New York Times*.
http://cityroom.blogs.nytimes.com/2010/08/21/stretch-laughter-yoga-serious-
benefits/

"Are You Meeting Your Laugh Quota? Why You Should Laugh Like a 5-Year-
Old." *Psychology Today*.
http://www.psychologytoday.com/blog/the-possibility-paradigm/201106/are-
you-meeting-your-laugh-quota-why-you-should-laugh-5-year-ol

"Study reveals laughter really is the best medicine." *BBC*.
http://www.bbc.co.uk/news/science-environment-14889165

"You'll Make It When You Fake It." *Psychology Today.*
http://www.psychologytoday.com/blog/codes-joy/201212/youll-make-It-when-you-fake-it

"Give Your Body a Boost—With Laughter." *WebMD.*
http://www.webmd.com/balance/features/give-your-body-boost-with-laughter

"7 Health Benefits of Laughter." *Gaiam Life.*
http://life.gaiam.com/article/7-benefits-laughter

"Happiness Model Could Help People Go from Good to Great." *Science Daily.*
http://www.sciencedaily.com/releases/2012/05/120507113742.htm

"What Makes Us Happy?" *Prevention.*
http://www.prevention.com/health/emotional-health/what-makes-us-happy

"Want to Be Happier? Here's How." *U.S. News & World Report.*
http://health.usnews.com/health-news/family-health/living-well/articles/2008/01/18/want-to-be-happier-heres-how

"10 Keys to True Happiness." *Reader's Digest.*
http://www.rd.com/health/wellness/10-keys-to-true-happiness/

"Connection & Happiness." *PBS.org.*
http://www.pbs.org/thisemotionallife/topic/connecting/connection-happiness

Brainy Quote.
http://www.brainyquote.com/quotes/topics/topic_humor.html#AUUHzFDQ7Av5iwEU.99

"Benefits of Moderate Sun Exposure." *Harvard Medical School Family Health Guide.*
http://www.health.harvard.edu/fhg/updates/update0604d.shtml

"Vitamin D." *MedlinePlus.*
http://www.nlm.nih.gov/medlineplus/ency/article/002405.htm

Chapter 10

"Media, Body Image, and Eating Disorders." *NEDA (National Eating Disorders Association).*
http://www.nationaleatingdisorders.org/media-body-image-and-eating-disorders

"Factors That May Contribute to Eating Disorders." *NEDA.*
http://www.nationaleatingdisorders.org/factors-may-contribute-eating-disorders

Brainy Quote.
http://www.brainyquote.com/quotes/keywords/love_yourself.html#kaqWSs9g
BHssJ2cF.99

"Role for a sense of self-worth in weight-loss treatments: helping patients develop self-efficacy." *PubMed.gov.*
http://www.ncbi.nlm.nih.gov/pubmed/18411382

"Self-efficacy as a predictor of weight change in African-American women." *PubMed.gov.*
http://www.ncbi.nlm.nih.gov/pubmed/15090632

Acknowledgments

From Jenn: Where to begin, where to begin. There are so many people who have supported and believed in me and this whole Fit Bottomed Girls mission from the beginning. Clearly, I have to thank Erin for joining me on this crazy ride—and setting out to save the world from "dieting" and deprivation. We basically share a brain; but I'm still astounded at how easy it is for us to write together. Almost like it was meant to be, huh? Who would have thought two girls giggling at their clumsiness in Zumba could do so much. Hard work and dedication pays off. And I'm honored to have you as a friend and business partner.

Then there's my husband Ryan, who has been my sounding board for so many ideas, issues, *everything else.* Truly a Fit Bottomed Dude, you are my rock, and you help me to dream even bigger. You make me a better person in every single way. And you're the best board of director that I know. And Siena? Thanks for opening package after package at FBG HQ—and being super cute in the process.

To my parents and all of my friends who have supported me through the writing and editing process, and are always interested in what I'm doing and genuinely gushing with pride, I am so grateful to have you in my life. Mom and Dad, you have given me so much, but your interest and support mean the most to me. I love you! Tish, you're my fellow FBG, best friend, soul mate. Can't wait until we go to the Oscars—Kiwi power! To my friends and the rest of my family, you know who you are, and you rock.

To all of those who have played a role in this book, holy moly, thank you! Zach Schisgal, thank you for seeing the potential in us and getting our message out there. You're truly a Fit Bottomed Girl at heart, which is the biggest compliment we can give a guy! To everyone at Random House, but especially Leah Miller and Mary Choteborsky, your direction and guidance have been paramount for fine-tuning our message and making this book a very practical guide for the everyday gal. You change lives! Sheryl, your brilliant help with the cover was priceless. (Not to mention that much of this book was written after either lunch with you or a workout at the Fit Pit—always a great way to get in a good headspace!)

A huge shout-out to those who have helped us build our brand from the beginning as well: Jim Wagner and Bob Lafferty at Lagom Design; Andrea Neasby-Porter, Shelton Koskie, and all of our writers (especially FBG Kristen!) past and present. And to all of the countless other firms and companies who have sponsored the site over the years, thanks for supporting FBG's mission!

Last but not least, a ginormous thank-you to all of the FBG, FBM, and FBE readers out there. Without you this wouldn't have been possible. So thanks for your gusto, honesty, humor, and inspiration. Keep on keeping a lid on the junk in the trunk—and having a damn good time doing it!

From Erin: So many people to thank, so little space. Jenn and I do share a brain, so on the book and business end, I'll just say "I concur; what she said. Thank you."

I must, of course, thank Jenn herself for taking me along for the FBG ride, being a constant source of healthy living inspiration, and being the most understanding and supportive friend and business partner. I couldn't have gotten this done without you (the thought of it gives me cold sweats) and your ambition, ideas, planning, and feedback. Thanks for being my twin and thinking for me when my brain is fried.

A monumental thanks to my husband, who has been a supporter of FBG from the beginning. I cannot fathom having written a single word without your support and the bit of extra sleep you let me have on the weekends. Thanks to my kiddos, Avery and Owen, who make me laugh every day and who give me much needed writing breaks by peeking over the baby gate into the office.

A big thanks, too, to the friends and family who allowed me to get work done by minding the kiddos—even if none of you could keep them from peeking over the baby gate into the office.

Index

Note: Page numbers in *italics* indicate recipes.